The Better Half of Life

The Better Half of Life

Jim Geddes

BROADMAN PRESS
Nashville, Tennessee

© Copyright 1987 • Broadman Press
All rights reserved
4257-32
ISBN: 0-8054-5732-1

Dewey Decimal Classification: 155.67
Subject Headings: AGING // MIDDLE AGE
Library of Congress Catalog Card Number: 87-8076
Printed in the United States of America

Library of Congress Cataloging-in-Publication Data

Geddes, Jim, 1935-
    The better half of life.

    1. Aging.   2. Middle age.   I. Title.
QP86.G38   1987   612'.67   87-8076
ISBN 0-8054-5732-1

The Aging Process

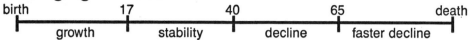

birth   17   40   65   death

growth   stability   decline   faster decline

Scientific View of The Life Span

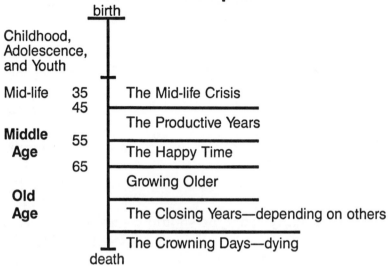

birth

Childhood, Adolescence, and Youth

Mid-life	35	The Mid-life Crisis
	45	The Productive Years
Middle Age	55	The Happy Time
	65	Growing Older
Old Age		The Closing Years—depending on others
		The Crowning Days—dying

death

Christian View of the Life Span

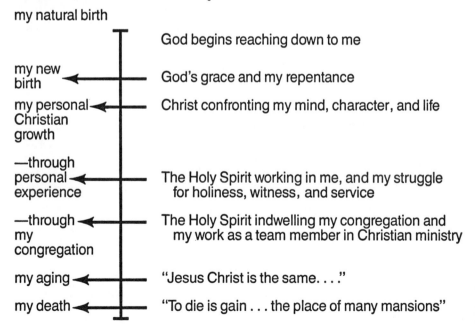

my natural birth

God begins reaching down to me

my new birth — God's grace and my repentance

my personal Christian growth — Christ confronting my mind, character, and life

—through personal experience — The Holy Spirit working in me, and my struggle for holiness, witness, and service

—through my congregation — The Holy Spirit indwelling my congregation and my work as a team member in Christian ministry

my aging — "Jesus Christ is the same. . . ."

my death — "To die is gain . . . the place of many mansions"

Quotations from the Past
About the Better Half of Life:

"The first thing is to acquire wisdom; gain understanding though it cost you all you have."

—Proverbs 4:7

Jesus said, "I have come that men may have life, and may have it in all its fullness."

—John 10:10*b*

"If a man lives for many years, he should rejoice in all of them."
—Ecclesiastes 11:8

"Grey hair is a crown of glory, and it is won by a virtuous life."
—Proverbs 16:31

"Grow old along with me!
The best is yet to be."
—Robert Browning

"Life is more delightful when it is on the downward slope."
—Seneca

Introduction

At last, in recent years, science has reversed itself and has corrected two major errors in its view of the aging process. There is now a new science of aging, and what a wave of optimism has resulted from the new science! How exciting it is to see a large segment of society rejuvenating itself, as so many mature and older adults are becoming more hopeful about their years ahead.

This is a book about the new science of aging and how it relates so well to Christian faith and practice. The aim of the book is to share with Christian people, workers with senior adults, and all senior adults, what the encouraging possibilities of the second half of life are. Let's dispel the gloom caused by so many years of false beliefs and wrong attitudes about aging.

The two major errors of science are considered in separate chapters in order to be certain they are ancient history, not present reality. First, the horrible myth of the twilight years is disproved. The second half of life is not a twilight zone of semidarkness and confusion and mental weakness. Science now says older persons actually know more, are wiser, and are more content. Second, the discouraging theory of disengagement has been set aside in favor of the activity theory. Older persons, according to the new theory, should engage in and pursue social activity and meaningful involvement in order to maximize their joy. They should not disengage but rather should keep mentally, physically, and socially active as fully as is practical and for as long as possible, if they would walk the pathway of lasting joy.

The Christian strategy of joy is studied, as are findings about longevity. In addition, there is a Christian overview of the life cycle.

The theme of the book is: Attitude is everything. The book's content has practical suggestions on how to have a realistic and positive Christian attitude in all six phases of the second half of life.

Is the second half of life better? This question is asked in several different chapters, and each chapter is intended to factually establish one or more ways that the second half of life is the better half.

This book is also an attempt to present the real body of factual information that exists today about all six phases of the second half of life. This is an exciting body of facts, and it points to many desirable conclusions which are evaluated from a Christian and biblical point of view.

Contents

Part I
The Aging Process

1

The Second Half Is Better!

Attitude Is Everything

There was once an amazing woman named Pat. "I'm *not* old," said Pat with a twinkle in her eye, "after all, I'm only seventy." What was amazing about her was that she almost always had that cheerful twinkle and a positive attitude, even if she had some pains and disappointments.

Pat had lived through a lifetime of personal disasters, yet she rarely complained and always had an encouraging word. Her troubles started at age six in first grade when her teacher belted Pat in the ear with a fist, resulting in ear abscesses and a series of major surgeries. School failure came next, followed by feelings of inferiority. Then came marital abuse and divorce, and more ill health, several serious car accidents, then death of family members. Finally, her friends and remaining family moved across the continent many miles away. It seemed, overall, as if disasters headed straight for Pat year after year, the way waves roll to the beach—one, then another, and another, and another. Pat shed many tears, but she kicked herself swiftly and fiercely whenever she came close to self-pity and negative thinking.

At age seventy there she was—a truly amazing and wonderful person—enjoying her old age. She was living alone in a small upstairs suite of a shabby apartment block with her TV, orange tabby cat, wheelchair, and a few albums of cherished family photos—but without spouse or family, without savings or pension, *and without legs!* That's right, no legs for Pat after one car accident. Her left leg had to be removed above the knee, and then the right leg when infection could not be controlled.

"Well, at least I have my arms and both hands, and a wheelchair and friends," says Pat. So she slides carefully from her bed onto the wheelchair and scoots around the suite and hallway, doing what she can and leaving the rest undone. She thoroughly enjoys whatever there is to enjoy and does not fret for long about her losses, disappointments, and unmet desires.

"It is a problem that we have no elevator in this old building, but I get someone to carry me and the chair down our three flights of stairs to the ground floor, and if I've saved any welfare money, I take a taxi to a shopping mall to shop around. Otherwise, I just sit by the ground floor entrance and look out at the street."

What has helped this survivor of countless disasters to keep a positive attitude, looking for new opportunities, enjoying whatever is at hand to enjoy, rarely pouting or complaining, and without even a trace of bitterness? Somehow she discounted the misfortunes of the past and placed great value on the enjoyments at hand. She refused to waste the "now" of her life by forever wishing that her past could have been different or better. The past—it was what it was, but it was over and gone. Instead, she savored every kind word from her neighbors in the today of her life. She enjoyed every laugh, relished every sip of tea, and counted the blessings that she was enjoying *today.* Tomorrow would have to take care of itself.

In a thoughtful moment she shared this pearl, born of her pains and disappointments but nourished by the reality of her faith in today: "You know, it took me the first forty years just to get an idea of who I am and what life is. Before forty I knew so little; I was making so many decisions and mistakes; I was in such a hurry that everything was a blur as I rushed along—thinking, planning, choosing, revising, correcting, experiencing, and regretting. It was a whirlwind of activity, and there were just enough misfortunes that I scarcely recovered from one before I was hit by the next one.

"Since age forty, I am slowly and surely learning how to live enjoyably. As I'm getting older, I think I'm getting wiser. This second half of my life—I mean the years after forty—it isn't perfect, but it certainly is the better half for me."

Lessons from Pat

1. Attitude is everything. Finances, relationships, even health are secondary. Do you need an attitude overhaul? Do you need to kick yourself and smarten up? The second half of life will have its share of frustrations and disappointments, but you should have learned by now that *attitude* goes a long way toward making the sky a beautiful blue. A positive attitude finds good in each hour of the day and makes us truly thankful for what we have.

And if this point isn't getting through to you, rent a wheelchair and an old shabby apartment for a week, and see how it all feels.

2. Are you forever wishing the past could have been different and better? Despair about the past is a hopeless dead end. Remember what is good about the good old days, and remember all the lessons of your mistakes. *Then* . . . forget the rest.

The present is what is important, and tomorrow should be on our minds, so we can seize its opportunities. Let the past stay where it is—behind you.

Have a Dream and Work to Make It Happen

Who is this old man walking in his cabbage patch in the warm sun on a warm and sunny Grecian hillside in the fourth century? He is the cabbage king, and he is humming a tune as he weeds and putters among his prizewinning cabbages. Why does he wear a purple-colored toga? To match his purple cabbages? While he is idling along the rows, a Roman general in full army regalia approaches respectfully and inquires of the old man's health. "Emperor, I bring you warmest greetings from your armies on the eastern front." "Justin, what a delight to see you, but the armies are no longer mine." "Sire, they wish you good health and long life, but they regret your retirement. Sire, would you resume your post? The empire needs you, for it never before had such a gifted leader and administrator."

The old man among the cabbages, one of Rome's greatest emperors, looks straight at the general. "Justin, my true friend and comrade, how do I appear to you? Do I look well? You used to tease me that I'm greying, balding, sagging, bulging here and there. You and I had many laughs about my weight, and you enjoyed teasing me about my big appetite. But Justin, how do I look?"

"Sire, you look rested, strong, and content. You look very alive and well."

"You answer well, Justin, for I truly am rested and content, after many years of struggle and exhausting work. I struggled to become emperor and then struggled to serve the empire well. But now I want to grow my cabbages on this hillside. I want to leave the problems and opportunities of the world to someone else."

"But Sire, your great talents of leadership and administration . . ."

"Wait, Justin, how good is your memory? Do you remember when I was with you leading the armies in the north, and I nearly drowned in that river crossing? I remember it well. As I was under the water and losing consciousness I thought that if I were to die right then, I would never live to retire in Greece and grow my cabbages, and I asked myself, for what was all my service and struggle if I couldn't enjoy my reward at the end? Justin, much of my sanity and survival in my years as emperor derived from the pleasure of anticipation of a well-deserved retirement. The cunning and treachery of my enemies, the obsequious fawning social climbers, the senators who were such pompous bores, the very real danger of the barbarian hordes on the borders of the empire, the finances and administration of the army and civil services—somehow I could survive this day by day knowing that there was a time coming when I would do new and different things in the second half of my life.

"Now, Justin, I am where I need to be, doing what I need to do, living my life on this hillside overlooking the sea, growing my cabbages. Can you accept my need to be here and do these things? I have a new friend, a peasant farmer, and he grows cabbages too. I enjoy his company. Next year he and I may import a different cabbage variety. And I have another new friend, a great cook, who prepares soups, stews, and salads "fit for an emperor." But I eat, not as emperor, but as a new friend. Justin, you can be my friend, too, but the emperor is no longer in me."

Lessons from the Cabbage King

1. Have a dream about what you would like your future to be, and work to make it happen. Plan your second half of life and do what you know you ought to be doing.

2. Life is process and change. Maturity is not the same as youth; maturity has new opportunities. Life moves on, and happiness comes when we let go of youth and all those things that block our enjoyment of the better half of life. See clearly the phases of the second half of life:

Age 35 to 45	Age 45 to 65	Age 65	Age 65 and the Final Years
Gradually letting go of youth and then seeing the new opportunities ahead.	Accepting the challenge of the empire and whatever, and giving your mind to your life work—enjoying the mind-set of of maturity and its broad understanding of being a person.	Gradually changing as we let go of some responsibilities, and then seeing the new opportunities ahead.	Accepting the challenge of being consultant, adviser, and friend, but insisting that the work and decisions shall involve others; accepting physical decline and enjoying the mental prime and wisdom of life.

3. Keep your sanity in the Responsibility Years, ages 45 to 65, by anticipating a change of pace and a change of focus after age 65. Then when the time comes, go ahead and make that change!— To consultant, adviser, friend, to cabbage grower, photographer, black Angus cattle breeder, traveler, participant in church and mission work or sports or playing the pipe organ, a more active

grandparent, or whatever is your choice, and even keeping a lesser hand in what was earlier your main line of endeavor.

4. Do not imagine that you can somehow enjoy the better half of life by the mentality and game plan, the focus and strategy of the first half of life. Each half requires its own rules. The better half needs better rules that develop the potential of the better half of life to its fullest.

First Half Rules "Striving"	Better Half Rules "Wisdom"
1. In your twenties and early thirties make beginnings —in developing a personal philosophy. —in marriage and parenting. —in vocation. —in hobbies and interests.	1. In your forties enrich your beginnings further —adding understanding and depth to your personal philosophy —adding understanding to your marriage and family and vocation.
2. Struggle, hurry, build, create, experiment, investigate, experience, acquire and develop knowledge and skills. *Mid-Life Rules*	2. Accept, adapt, understand, comprehend, interrelate, integrate, synthesize, acquire wisdom, and know yourself.
3. In your late thirties begin to enrich your beginnings by adding depth and understanding to your personal philosophy and your interpersonal relationships.	3. In your fifties begin again! Make new beginnings! —Make one new friend every year. —Take on new projects that are worthy of a wise person. —Build toward a great worthwhileness of your own life which will peak in your sixties and seventies, and which will endure to the end.

Toward Wisdom

What are the opportunities after forty? How should each person grow and mature so that all the years after forty are a swelling crescendo and a crowning achievement in the fifties, sixties, seventies, and beyond?

Eula just knew in her thirties that the death of her Texas pastor-husband could not be the end for her. Could she live without the husband for whom she had had a consuming passion and pride? "Wrong question," said Eula, "of course I can live without the great love of my life, but not without a year of tears. I have no choice in the matter. The Lord gave, the Lord took away. It will take me time, but I must look ahead and rebuild my life." And so she did, raising her four children on a church secretary's salary, devoting her life to being the best person she could be, and earning the respect and love of all who knew her because of her energy, dedication, and cheerfulness. But it was in her years after forty that she made a number of right decisions that kept her life building in quality and adventure.

Age 44—decision to remain single (she felt this was best for her), in order to give herself to family and church.

Age 51—decision to change employment to bookkeeper, to help in her son's business.

Age 60—decision to retire early and help in her congregation, and what a helper she was!

Age 62—decision to move to Africa to live with her daughter and help in a village mission station in Tanzania.

Eula's wisdom taught her to walk firmly in Christian faith daily and not to become too wrapped up in setbacks and disappointments. "Live for the next minute, and that is fifty-nine seconds too long. When problems are pressing, pray, get a good night's sleep and a good breakfast, and then you will find your solution." Eula lived fully right to the day of her death.

Jack invested his twenties and thirties in mastering the facts and skills of his profession, and at age forty, that was all he had: a mass of facts and skills. In the five years age forty to forty-five, he learned to take many of the facts and put them together in a meaningful way. In the years from age forty-six to age fifty-eight (when he retired), he was able to apply the facts and skills wisely to the great benefit of his clients. But from age fifty-eight (retirement) to his death at age seventy-seven, he had the greatest enjoyment and satisfaction of his life as he consulted on a part-time basis with young professionals in their twenties and thirties who still did not have it all together in a meaningful way. The years

after forty: What should they mean? For this professional person
the formula was:

$$\underset{\text{(in profession)}}{\text{WISDOM}} \quad + \quad \underset{\text{(scaled down to part time)}}{\text{OPPORTUNITY}} \quad = \quad \underset{\text{(in second half)}}{\text{SATISFACTION}}$$

Jack, like many of us, found that the years after forty took a
sharp turn for the better when the express train of life slowed
down enough that he could look out the train window and see the
scenery clearly for the first time as the train moved by at a slower
pace. *Slow down, if you want to see meaning and purpose.* The
better half of life is all about meaning and purpose which we learn
by *slowing down in order to see better.*

Larry and Mabel have been married many years and now are
in their mid-seventies. In their twenties and thirties each one was
always right even though they often disagreed, and each one's
loyalty to his or her ideals often produced yelling, tears, confusion, and bitterness. Compromise was not their style. Patience
and dialogue were in short supply. However, he was the great love
of her life, and she was the great love of his life, and slowly, at
times painfully, they worked toward a deeper understanding and
acceptance of each other. This started in their forties, improved
in their fifties, and blossomed in their sixties and seventies.

Love birds in old age: What is surprising about that? After all,
shouldn't everything about relationships get better with age if we
are working well on personal growth and understanding?

Their marriage began to improve when they were in their mid-
forties and Mabel said to herself, "Why am I taking his weaknesses personally? Why don't I enjoy the good in him and try to
live with the rest?"

As Mabel was saying this to herself, Larry was beginning to say
to himself, "Even if I am the one who is right, what enjoyment is
there in being right and being alone? After all, I have faults, so
why shouldn't Mabel have the right to hers? She is good in so
many other ways; why am I picking up on every little flaw?

Lesson from Larry and Mabel

The first half of life is often focused on getting the facts straight, but the better half of life takes the facts, in all their complexity, and relates them meaningfully together so that we get the broad perspective. "Don't miss the forest for the trees" is the message in the second half.

Sour Second Halves

Sometimes, tragically, the second half turns sour. Instead of being the better half, the second half *in a minority of people* fails to blossom, stumbles, falters along with much difficulty, edging toward despair.

How could Basil know that his proper, formal British politeness and emotional inhibition would cause his fifties to be lonely, as old friends preferred more enthusiastic and spontaneous company? Fortunately, in his early sixties a professional colleague set him straight, and Basil was able to relish the taste of joy in his old age.

Adelaide wasn't as fortunate as Basil. In her forties and fifties, she refused to let go of her youth. "You are as young as you feel—nothing has really changed," dreamed Adelaide as she panicked at every new wrinkle and extra patch of gray hair and exercised and dieted with greater determination than ever. In her sixties she was forever wishing her past could have been different. It was easy to see she had never really planned to grow old, and she had no idea of the opportunities and delights involved in leaving youth behind. For Adelaide the second half of life was a pitiful unfortunate appendage attached to the end of youth. In her view one didn't accept old age; one fought it or denied its existence. No one came along to help her see anything differently, and the second half was sour.

As great a completion and fulfillment as the second half of life is intended to be, it is true that the second half of life can be soured at times by:

1. False beliefs about the second half of life.
2. Wrong values about the second half of life.

Let us list some false beliefs and wrong values that usually cause life to go sour. Then alongside these false beliefs and wrong values, let us list plainly what are the true beliefs and right values that usually improve the second half of life.

Beliefs About the Second Half of Life

False Beliefs

True Beliefs

1. In the second half of life the human brain becomes weak and ineffective, and we slip into the twilight zone of confusion and forgetting.

1. In the second half of life we sometimes do forget the trivial and the unimportant, but experience helps us to reason better about the great issues of life.

2. Slowing down means less satisfaction and joy.

2. Slowing down leads to much deeper understanding and contentment. At last we see the real meaning.

3. Retirement is the end of feeling useful.

3. The truth is that retirement is a great opportunity to get rid of unwanted roles and to accept vital new ones.

4. Sex is for youth.

4. Sexual interest and enjoyment never dies, and love goes on building as long as we keep on building it.

5. You can't make good friends in middle age and old age.

5. In middle age and old age we finally understand what friendship is, and we should aim to make one new friend a year.

6. You can't take on new roles and new responsibilities in middle age and old age.

6. New roles and new responsibilities are forever the spice of life, and we should find new roles every year as long as we live.

Values About the Second Half of Life

Wrong Values

Right Values

1. Worth is youth.

1. Worth is worth, wherever you find it, and is more likely in middle age and old age than in the instability, inexperience, and haste of youth.

2. You will be happier in old age by accepting the inevitable and becoming relatively socially inactive.

2. You will be happier in old age if you struggle to keep as active socially as you would like to be.

3. More means better.

3. Usually less food is better, and more enjoyable, as we learn the art

Wrong Values	Right Values
	of savoring every morsel. Less money is often more enjoyable. Less strength of body can be irrelevant beside more strength of mind.
4. Beauty means no wrinkles, no bulging, no graying, no sagging.	4. Beauty is goodness, purpose, faith, meaning, and joy.

A Christian Views the Second Half

God has *not* decreed that our second half of life will automatically be the better half. He does *not* guarantee that the quality of life will improve as we grow older, nor does He guarantee that we will all get wiser with each passing year. But He does give all of us this opportunity to work to make our life what it ought to be year by year. To the Christian, life is learning to walk with God, and wisdom is obedience to God's commands. As we grow older, we ought to come to know more about life, more about God, and more about how to know and enjoy God's purpose and plan. The more we walk with Him, the closer we ought to be to Him. Therefore, life should get better and better—if we are learning and if we are finding true wisdom.

But it is *tuum est*—very much *up to ourselves*—what we do with each day and whether in fact life gets better or worse or drags along at the same level.

God does offer to everyone the formula:

FAITH AND REASON→ OBEDIENCE →WISDOM →MAXIMUM FULFILLMENT

It is our choice of whether or not to accept the formula.

There are two special reasons why the second half of life should be exciting and precious to the true Christian. First, there is satisfaction in aging because with every passing day we know we

are one more day older and one day closer to our own death and
liberation into God's eternal presence. The Christian learns to
await the great day of life's consummation with patience and
anticipation, not with dread nor fear. True believers are like pris-
oners in their cells marking on their wall calendars the days
remaining to their release to freedom. The second half is better
just because it is closer to the complete and final freedom of God's
eternal presence.

The second reason why the second half of life is exciting and
satisfying to the believer is Christian service. We are finally getting wise enough after forty to know how to enhance and promote
the noble and worthy projects of our life and of the kingdom of
God on earth. An example of a great project of the Kingdom is any
New Testament congregation that takes its responsibilities seriously. No wonder there are so many happy older persons who find
much fulfillment as they enjoy the Spirit's abiding Presence in
their congregation. What an excitement to be part of a New Testament congregation.

Another example of a thrilling project of the Kingdom is Bold
Mission Thrust. How many millions of persons of all ages will
catch the excitement and adventure of this Kingdom project. Bold
Mission Thrust is a true life changer, life builder, and life winner.

Hope is the confidence that God is in all of my tomorrows. Hope
is another reason that Christian people should find the second
half of life exciting. Hope is a reason to be optimistic about the
years ahead. Hope is a challenge to fill those coming years with
worthwhile projects. Stop worrying about what tomorrow holds if
you know who holds tomorrow. God holds the tomorrows; God
holds your tomorrow. Can you have confidence in Him? Can you
believe He will hold you together in one piece in the remaining
years of your life, developing and building your life toward a
consummation and crowning at the great transition day?

Finally, a word about joy. Joy comes in different ways to each
individual, but the Christian's joy has some common features
which precede it:

1. We are joyful when we know we are making progress to become the Christian person we ought to be.

2. We are joyful when we know we are investing our lives in the best possible way in Christian service.

3. We are joyful when we take steps to change what needs to be changed in our selves and in our life situations.

4. We are joyful when we refuse to become preoccupied with the discomforts, frustrations, and disappointments of our daily lives.

As we consider the full meaning and implications of these four prerequisites of joy, we see the second half of life becomes joyful only as we make progress in our individual development. Joy comes when we are making basic progress in living, and it is a reward for making the right decisions based on sound values. We ought not to pursue joy, but joy will come as we pursue its prerequisites.

Making the Best of the Second Half

The evidence of science, the wisdom of religion, and the testimony of personal experience—all three of these sources favor the second half as the better half of life. They provide different types of information, but together they give strong support for the potential of joy in all the years after forty. So far, we have been looking at personal evidence of older persons. We have also introduced some Christian evidence. Much of the remaining evidence about the better half of life is comprehensive scientific research, and the conclusions of this research will be presented in the chapters ahead. These conclusions of science form an amazing parallel with the truths of the Scripture, and together they identify some important principles and guidelines about how to obtain the greatest happiness and peace of mind in all the years after forty.

What are these principles and guidelines for the years after forty? Let us outline here in short form the basic principles and guidelines to be discussed:

1. *Pursue virtue, wisdom, and noble adventures.* There is a fundamental basic emotion of joy. True joy comes, after age forty, from the pursuits of virtue, wisdom, and noble adventures. If you

want joy, do not pursue it, or it will evade you. Instead, pursue the prerequisites of joy: virtue, wisdom, and noble adventures.

2. *Improve with age.* As it slows down, the body actually begins to do many things better, but it is *the mind* of a person over age forty that really makes the second half better.

3. *Old bodies are often better*—slower but better. The human body after age forty is capable of continuous hard work without wearing out, and it has a much better mixture of hormones for enjoying life. The enemy of old bodies is *not age but inactivity.* Lesser enemies are excess weight, hypertension, ineffective worry, disease, alcohol, and nicotine abuse.

4. *Old brains are better*—slower but better. Intelligence does not decline with age in healthy, active persons unless there is mental inactivity, hypertension, or disease. Intellectual decline in older persons is reversible through moderate mental exercise and stimulation and/or medical treatment of hypertension and disease. Older persons are much wiser, as a rule, and they know more than younger persons. But older persons do wish more time to analyze a situation before proceeding.

5. *The second half of life is two stages, not one.*

   a. Middle Adulthood—ages forty-five to sixty-five. This is a period of *moderate decline* of physical strength and energy, combined with maximum intellectual capacity. Wisdom usually makes a good beginning in middle adulthood, though it begins in youth in a small number of persons.

   b. Older Adulthood—age sixty-five and up. This is a period of faster decline in physical strength, combined with intellectual strength and maximum wisdom.

   Individuals do not always fit into their chronological age group. Individuals may be biologically up to twenty years older or up to twenty years younger than their chronological age because of life-style and heredity.

6. *Mid-Life Crisis.* Both males and females frequently experience a crisis of awareness of aging, usually in the late thirties or early forties.

Every mid-life crisis is an opportunity for self-analysis and revision and refinement of life goals, expectations, and hopes. Mid-life crises are usually nature's shock therapy to get us to let go of youth and to welcome maturity.

7. *The Productive Years—ages forty-five to fifty-five.* Many in their forties experience a sharp life turn for the better, marked by increased deeper understanding of both self and others. This is when wisdom often makes its first strong appearance, viewed as an ability to use our skills and knowledge with understanding and good judgment.

8. *The Happy Time—ages fifty-five to sixty-five.* The happy time —the happiest decade in the life cycle—is the period from age fifty-five to age sixty-five. However, the years before age fifty-five and after age sixty-five are also rich in contentment and fulfill-ment because we are at last coming to understand what it is to be a person and how to fit in to the scheme of things. We finally know, in our fifties, how to do good with discretion so that it does not turn sour. We have an accuracy, perception, and insight that solves problems before they begin. We have the mental resources to know what to accept and what to change. We push at the right times, and we know when to back off. Trial and error have been replaced with wisdom in most matters. This is the prime of life, lasting well into the sixties and seventies, and for some, into the eighties and nineties.

9. *Growing Older—age sixty-five and up.* These persons are the survivors. They have survived wars, disease, and accidents. They are the ones who have outlived peers, spouses, siblings, and friends. They usually understand their good fortune to be alive in whatever shape, and they count on being here at least for tomor-row to experience, enjoy, and shape their own lives and the lives of others. They cultivate joy, they share wisdom, and they keep as active as possible. They have usually worked successfully through despair. They have come to terms with dying and death, but their interest is in living and supporting whatever they cher-ish, including family, ideals, and causes.

10. *Growing Older with a Positive Outlook.* Only in the years after sixty can we view the life span from a personal perspective.

What an advantage! We really know what life is all about—what is important and what is unimportant, what is a big issue and what is a small issue. A mature attitude helps to lift us above conflicts and disappointments and to see these as part of a bigger picture and part of a total situation. It is the attitude we bring to a situation or relationship that counts the most. The best attitude grows out of true beliefs, sound values, and reasonable expectations. No wonder those over sixty have better attitudes, tempered as they are by many years of rich experiences of living. Better attitudes are essential to make the best of the better half of life.

Four negatives—depression, anxiety, loneliness, and boredom —turn out to be positives, if we face them honestly and make needed changes in our life.

11. *The Closing Years.* There is a brief period of physical weakness and dependence on family or nursing care, when it is no longer wise to live alone. Either we move in with family, or we move toward nursing care. We need to make the choice. Gratitude and relief are genuine when older persons receive the help they know they need.

A beautiful part of the closing years is the high-risk living and challenge that comes with the desire to be as active and responsible as possible. Granted, we cannot do as much, but let us do all that we can, whenever we can. Out of this desire to be active and responsible come many expressions of goodness, courage, and hope.

12. *The Crowning Days.* Dying and the meaning of life. The final few days and weeks ought to be a crowning and summation of life. The crowning is, of course, done by others, and represents a recognition of the uniqueness and value of one human life, appreciated for its meaning and its contribution. It is not selfish praise, but it is a thank you and a final tribute. This is the time for others to say it all—to the person being crowned.

The final days are brief as we wind up and settle our stewardship, weaving together the last loose strands into the finished fabric or tapestry of one life. We accept God's sovereignty over all of life, and we are ready to accept His decision about the day of our death. There is then a little more waiting, but we are ready—ready to close this chapter and start again on the other side. O the rest that is coming soon! And then it comes.

2

A Strategy of Joy

The scientific and Christian strategies for joyful living are at last compatible, since science has reversed itself on several major points. What are these two strategies, and how can they now be blended together as one strategy of joy? Let us first look at the scientific views, and then let us describe the Christian view. By way of introduction, we can state that maximum joy in the second half of life comes from:

1. A strategy or plan of action that includes meaningful ongoing responsibilities, activities, and roles that will last throughout the life span.

2. Realism and hope about the opportunities of middle adulthood, later adulthood, and the closing years.

3. True beliefs, sound values, and good attitudes about the meaning and purpose of human life.

Don't Disengage!

Modern scientists do not agree on the proper pathway to joy. Some say that the disengaged person is the happy person. They define disengagement as a natural and normal process of middle and older adulthood in which we as individuals begin naturally to withdraw from social activities and social involvement, and society naturally withdraws from us. To find maximum joy in the second half of life, we should, according to this view, accept reduced social and interpersonal interactions as inevitable. By going along with this natural process we will be happier. Accept the inevitable and become relatively socially inactive. Disengage! Let go of your roles, responsibilities, and commitments, as this is the road to greatest happiness in the second half of life.

While this disengagement theory is not a popular one among gerontologists, it does have some truth to it. Many older persons are making the mistake of trying to hang on to youthful activities and maintain the high-speed pace of those in their twenties and thirties. These persons should disengage *from high gear*—not get out of the race altogether, but switch *to a lower gear.* The disengagement theory goes too far in advocating withdrawal; but it is correct, if we can revise its message slightly, in advising those over age forty that life is a new ball game with rules that will change every five to ten years for the remainder of life. The second half is better when we stop pretending we are "twenty-nine and holding." The disengagement theory is partially correct if we can interpret it to mean: not disengage, but slow down, not withdraw from society but gradually alter and reduce our intense interpersonal commitments. Act your age, and there are age-appropriate activities! Being the world's oldest teenager is not the road to joyful living.

Keep Active!

Modern scientific research has not confirmed the disengagement theory. Rather, it has confirmed the opposite view, namely that joy after age forty goes with *activity,* not with disengagement. You will be happier by struggling to keep socially active. Granted, there is physical decline and increasing weakness, but don't accept your decline passively: Fight it. The activity theory says it is society that wants to withdraw from the individual against his or her wishes. An individual will be happier if he opposes those social forces that are withdrawing from him. Activity is the elixir of youth. Don't worry about wearing out because rusting out through inactivity is the much greater danger. Don't sit staring at the TV or out the window. Fill your life with meaningful activity.

Reduce Your Interpersonal Commitments

A team of researchers, Maddox and Eisdorfer, provide evidence in favor of activity theory and against disengagement theory. They prove there is a positive relation between activity and morale. The active persons are the happier ones.

However, these researchers also found that as age increases (from age sixty upward), the total sum of activity may decline without affecting the joy of living. We do need to keep socially active and socially involved, but we will be gradually reducing the level of activity as life progresses into later adulthood and the final years.

Maddox states there are two types of activity: interpersonal and noninterpersonal. Aging should result in a reduction of interpersonal activity (intense personal and emotional involvements), and this reduction will not result in any loss of the joy of living. But aging should not result in reduction of noninterpersonal activity (social, recreational, political, and religious commitments). It is wrong strategy to reduce these noninterpersonal activities in later adulthood; morale suffers in direct proportion to this reduction in noninterpersonal activity (social, religious, etc.).

Go ahead and allow some interpersonal disengagement, but fight to maintain your noninterpersonal activities every step of the way because these activities are great contributors to the joy of living. Be active all your life in your congregation, the Legion, the Eastern Star, your professional association, or your vocational association. Get out of the house often, whatever your age, provided health safety allows it.

Keep your garden going all your life, but let it get smaller. Do whatever you wish, and do, as long as you have the strength to do it. Get there on your own two feet or with a cane or with crutches or with a wheelchair, but at least get there. Be a doer—talk, listen, garden, read, bake, travel, clean house, write, sing, teach, repair, mend, plan, think, agree and disagree, laugh and mourn, create, discover, learn, plan, harvest, build, rebuild, paint, decorate, visit, pray, share, study, walk, stand, and exercise.

Be a doer of things you will enjoy. Pat cleaned her suite, talked to friends, went to the shopping mall in her wheelchair. Jack shared his wisdom of his profession. Eula served the Lord in her congregation, and then went to Africa to a village mission station. Each of us needs to find those noninterpersonal activities—social, recreational, political, religious—that bring us joy. Recent research on the human life span shows that the vast majority of people are healthy and happy in their seventies, eighties, and nineties, and an even greater majority would be happy if they would change their gloomy expectations about the second half of life and become more active.

Find New Roles and New Responsibilities
Role-exit theory is our third and final modern scientific theory about finding joy in the second half of life. Roles are important because they foster activity. The role-exit theory is one special aspect of activity theory, demonstrating *how to keep active* in the second half. Roles tend to exit for many persons, and if they do, they should be replaced with new roles. New roles bring new activities. If we have no roles, we are often staring out the window with nothing enjoyable to do.

There are many fortunate and unfortunate examples of role-exit, and these examples reveal *some principles* about roles and activity in the second half of life.

Roles are for individuals. One person's ecstasy is another person's boredom. One person's role satisfaction is another's disaster. Roles are for individuals, and each of us must find his or her own roles that will maximize the joy of life. Georgia was a good cook who hated cooking! Heaven for her was hiring a cook to do the Christmas baking. She would rather clean barns, garden, milk cows, or do any sort of outside work. So Georgia found her own heaven in her middle age and older adulthood by being a good customer at the local bakery and by keeping a prize-winning garden. What is your cup of tea? Baking or gardening? Take your pick and enjoy (en-joy) yourself.

Some older individuals enjoy many roles in their second half of life. Brian was an appliance repairman but retired early to enjoy many roles and activities. In his fifties, sixties, and seventies, he enjoyed himself. His family and friends enjoyed him. He was always busy in a wide variety of roles including:

1. Family member.
2. Friend.
3. Church member and Christian helper. (He helped in construction of three buildings for congregational worship and education.)
4. Cook. (Who could brown a better gravy or make better cabbage rolls or a tastier apple pie?) He even helped occasionally in his daughter's restaurant.
5. Grower of strawberries—by the barrel.
6. Appliance repair—for neighbors and friends.
7. Sports fisherman.
8. Avid fan of professional sports.

He was energetic, busy, and contented—right to his final day in his eighties.

By comparison, Brian's younger brother Cyril had no interests and no roles except complainer, criticizer, and alcohol abuser. Cyril thought Brian's cooking and church work were senseless, but Cyril never found his own roles and activities that should have become his own pathway to joy in the second half of life.

First-half hobbies can become second-half delights. The assembly line worker had always enjoyed photography. And in the second half of her life, photography filled the bill for a new role. She had her own darkroom and took and developed her own pictures for weddings and other events.

A pastor-and-wife team retired and taught Greek in Tanzania in a seminary, but only one year out of every three, coming home for the other two years. Their fee for teaching was only travel and accommodation. During his ministry as pastor he had always had a passion for the Greek language. His wife's passion had always been travel and being a friend. Now, in their second half of life, their first-half passions became the key to second-half delights.

The homemaker always enjoyed volunteer service in her youth, working in a small coffee shop in an office building. In her forties she purchased the coffee shop and kept it running very well on a small scale. She moved the coffee shop only once to another office building when in her sixties, and she kept on running it well into her seventies, coming in each morning with her granddaughter at 9:30 AM and closing up at 3:30 PM. She was first and foremost the homemaker and family person, but she always enjoyed (en-joy-ed) *her* coffee shop. Do you have an old first-half hobby that might, with effort, become your second-half delight?

Some roles do not exit; they shrink. Remember Jack, who became a professional consultant part-time in his sixties and seventies, still following the main line of his career, but on a reduced scale. Similar masterpieces of second-half living are Alex and Fae, who kept their hand in ranching in their later years. Their daughters and son operated the family business, but Dad and Mom had a few cattle of their own and helped around the ranch on a reduced scale. In her mid-eighties Fae enjoyed her garden, cooking, her grandchildren, and all the family talk about plans for expanding the ranch. In the worst of winter Alex and Fae are away from the ranch in south Texas, but early in spring they head back north and west, and Alex is excited about his minor roles on the ranch for spring, summer, and fall. In their final years they have set aside their plans to move away to senior citizen housing, mainly because they love knowing they are helpful on the ranch; also, they love their small house on the ranch and the other houses and families that occupy the other corners of the ranch yard. Especially, they love to see their grandchildren dropped off each day at the ranch by the school bus. How fast the children are growing! How they gobble up Fae's baking! What could possibly be more joyful than this contentment and sense of purpose in the crown and summation of their lives?

Brand-new roles can be a source of joy. Consider Fraser, who, on the day of his retirement, went briefly to visit his daughter and son-in-law, planning to return to Scotland after the visit and sit back, put his feet up, and enjoy the leisure of rest and inactivity. For years Fraser had relished this vision of his retirement. After so many years of do, do, and do more, how great it would be to sit back and do *nothing!* Oh, what a rest it would be!

But fate smiled on Fraser and saved him from this slow death of nothingness when he met old Robertson, the son-in-law's father. Old Robertson, long retired, filled every day doing as much as he could without overdoing it. He didn't sit around; he got up when he was ready and went to the stock exchange, then off to lunch with friends, then home early to wife and family and such social, religious, and recreational activities as he enjoyed.

Fraser was dumbfounded at old Robertson's different view of the second half of life, but he returned to Scotland and did the right thing by taking a part-time job ten to two Monday to Friday at a service station two blocks away. His job? Cleaning cars, waiting on customers at the cash register, and helping in any way he could. Fraser joyfully held this job for seven years from age sixty-five to age seventy-two, after which he took a different job that he is enjoying still. What powerful evidence that brand-new roles can be a source of joy in the second half of life.

"I have never done that sort of thing before, but I would be glad to try it now"—those are the right words to begin new challenges in the second half of life. Be a Fraser and try something new, because new roles can bring joy.

A Christian Strategy of Joy

We have been looking at the scientific conclusions on how to find satisfaction in the second half of life. Stated briefly, these are:

A. Don't disengage from life, but let go of youth. Accept a reduction of your interpersonal, emotional commitments and involvement.

B. Keep as active as you can, physically and mentally throughout the life span.

C. When old familiar roles exit or shrink, be sure to replace them with new roles aimed at maintaining social, religious, and recreational activity.

This is the sum of science concerning the attainment of joy.
Is there nothing more to be said of joy? Has science said it all?

Science is helpful, and we should learn as much as we can from it, but science is merely a useful introduction to a much greater strategy of joy for second-half living that is based on Christian faith. The Christian view of the second half of life includes a magnificent strategy of joy, which deserves to be considered in detail.

True joy begins with awareness of God's great love for us. How does true and lasting joy begin? This joy begins with the discovery that the Eternal God is a person who is loving and kind, and He has a purpose and meaning for every life. Joy comes when we respond to God's love by genuine repentance, which is a change of heart and mind toward God. Repentance, in turn, brings the joy of forgiveness and the joy of the friendship and fellowship of God. Then from His forgiveness and friendship, we receive that illumination that helps us pursue our own destiny and His purposes for us. "[His] wonderful purposes are all for our good" (Ps. 40:5). "God is love" (1 John 4:10). "Christ died for us while we were yet sinners, and that is God's own proof of his love towards us" (Rom. 5:8). "God loved the world so much that he gave us his only Son" (John 3:16). Jesus says, "I have come that men may have *life,* and may have it in all its fullness" (John 10:10, author's italics). "I wish you all joy in the Lord, I will say it again: all joy be yours" (Phil. 4:4).

If you want joy, respond to God's love and grace! The second half of life is much better when we use time to reexamine and strengthen the foundations of faith. What a surprise and joy for us as we discover that our mature minds can now appreciate God's wisdom and purpose much better than our youthful mind ever could before.

Religious faith is a solid source of joy in the second half of life.

Christian joy increases with age! Christian joy is like a mathematical progression which grows and develops as the years go by.

"If a man lives for many years, he should rejoice in all of them" (Eccl. 11:8). Middle age and old age should be times of excitement and rejoicing because we are at last learning how to follow in Christ's footsteps. Christian joy is properly a crescendo which reaches its full strength in the second half of life. Joy requires time to grow, but if given time, joy grows, comes to bud, and then to full blossom, without ever fading. Joy in our final years is a natural consequence of faithful Christian living.

No wonder Paul's final prison letters, in the last months of his life, are epistles of joy. That is how it ought to be: our finding full joy in the final years.

Another example is Buck, a survivor of World War I, who served the Lord for a lifetime minus one arm and one leg. Buck's joy expanded in his second half of life. He was getting himself figured out and shaped up and finally knew much more about how to live joyfully. Three things among others brought joy to Buck and his wife Rachel.

1. Share your wisdom with the young.
2. Ask for and accept help from the young.
3. Invite the young to share a meal.

Buck and Rachel handled these three things skillfully, and their lives were more active and more joyful as a result.

If you want joy, do not pursue it! The New Testament Christians of the first century, as well as the New Testament Christians of today, knew that it is not best to pursue joy but to let it come to us. True joy cannot be seized; it has to be earned as we pursue the full potential of a Christian life. By walking forward patiently and confidently in the pursuit of personal excellence and by striving to be the best possible Christians, we obtain joy as a reward. Joy is a reward for success in the pursuit of God's purpose. Joy is a spin-off of faithfulness in the Christian walk. Joy is a side effect, not a goal, and it only comes, in its fullness, to those who do not pursue it but who, instead, pursue the threefold goals of Christian living: virtue, wisdom, and noble adventure.

If you want joy, pursue virtue. Pursue virtue in the second half, and you will obtain joy as well as virtue. "Gray hair is a crown of glory, and it is won by a virtuous life" (Prov. 16:31). Notice the biblical view that gray hair (the second half of life) is a crown of great honor, not a pitiful, withering weakness. Notice also that the crown is won by virtue (sound values, and strong conscience and self-control). Virtue is pivotal if the second half of life is to become the better half. Virtue is the proper emphasis for the second half, and second-half persons should work at virtue.

Virtue includes Godliness and keeping the Commandments. The Deuteronomic principle of Moses makes blessing and joy dependent on virtue and obedience to God's commands!

"Keep his statutes and commandments . . . then all will be well with you . . . and you will live long" (Deut. 4:40).

"Conform to all the Lord your God commands you, if you would live and prosper" (Deut. 5:33).

"If you listen, O Israel, and are careful to observe [the commandments], you will prosper and increase greatly" (Deut. 6:3).

"Do what is right and good in the Lord's eyes so that all may go well with you" (Deut. 6:18).

"If you listen to these laws . . . then the Lord . . . will love you, [and] bless you" (Deut. 7:13).

Remember that virtue is the goal, and virtue includes sound values and strong conscience, self-control, and maturity. Pursue virtue, and joy will come to you as well.

If you want joy, pursue wisdom. Pursue wisdom, and joy will come to you as well. Wisdom is a state of mind that includes sound judgment, patience, and insight. Wisdom resolves problems. Wisdom turns problems into opportunities. Wisdom takes the broad look, and wisdom leads eventually to joy.

Wisdom is God's gift to those who are walking in His direction.

"The Lord bestows wisdom/and teaches knowledge and understanding" (Prov. 2:6).

"If any of you falls short in wisdom, he should ask God for it" (Jas. 1:5).

"The first thing is to acquire wisdom;/gain understanding though it cost you all you have" (Prov. 4:7).

Wisdom is a priority on the pathway to joy. Seek wisdom.

Pursue noble and worthwhile adventures, and joy will come to you as well. These adventures are great projects that give expression to your highest ideals. They are battles you believe need to be fought. They are major investments of your energy and skills in any worthwhile endeavors that represent your own values and beliefs. The Christian strategy of joy is to invest your life in the service of Him whom you believe, by giving full support in a Christian manner to family, congregation, community, and country. If you want abundant spin-offs of joy, invest your life in the promotion of things you believe are most important. Lose your life in the service of a great cause, and joy will be the return on your investment. One example of a noble adventure is Bold Mission Thrust: a massive effort to spread the gospel and develop a worldwide network of cooperating coordinated New Testament congregations.

3

A Longer, Healthier, Better Half of Life

Does "Longer Life" Mean "Better Life"?

We all know a few second-half losers who, because of wrong attitudes, are miserable, unhappy, and only rarely experience joy. These older people are sure proof that longer life does not necessarily mean happiness and joy. But in spite of this miserable minority, the second half does have superb potential for joy. Because of this second half potential for joy, listen to science to see how to extend the second half—to make it longer and to make it healthier. This information, when added to the strategy of joy which we have just discussed at length, means that the second half certainly ought to be better as well as longer.

However, the desire to extend the length of life is not a search for the elixir of youth. Eternal youth is *not* the goal. Learn to be glad that youth is over with all of its haste, inexperience, and trial-and-error learning. Youth is gone; let it go. Our goal now is to learn to extend our second half, not to extend our youth. Maturity is much to be preferred over youth, and maturity is the heart of second-half living. Finally, remember that "second half" does not mean "second class." Second half ought to mean first-class living. Let's work to make the second half the better half of life.

Theories of Aging

The "Wear and Tear" Theory. This theory notes that there is both death and decline in function of nondividing cells of vital organs. The number of healthy brain and liver cells is steadily declining from birth, and aging is the inefficiency that comes from having fewer and fewer of these nondividing cells with which to maintain vital life functions. The reduced number of these nondividing cells begins to have a noticeable and measurable effect by age twenty-five. By age seventy loss of brain neurons in the healthy brain is an accumulated 44 percent. From age thirty to age seventy loss of functional glomeruli (kidney cells) is a total of 56 percent. The similar loss of functional cells in aging lungs results in decreased elasticity of lungs and reduction of maximum breathing capacity by 57 percent (and an 80 percent reduction in smokers). Cardiac output decreases 30 percent from age thirty to age seventy. Muscle strength decreases 45 percent from age thirty to age seventy. A healthy seventy-year-old functions only 15 percent as well as a thirty-year-old when doing sustained heavy work. We age and die, according to this theory, because the vital organs become less and less efficient, less and less able to deal with infection, trauma, and other stressful conditions.

However, because of different life-styles we do not all age at the same rate. Twenty percent of all twenty-five-year-olds are already biologically age forty because of a life-style that speeds up the aging process. Also, twenty percent of all forty-year-olds are biologically only age twenty-five because their life-style slows down degenerative processes. In our next theme of this chapter, under the heading "Ten Commandments for a Longer Life," we list those factors which slow down the aging process.

Immunity Theory. This view notes that people do not just die of old age; rather, they die from infection and malfunction of at least one vital body system, whether heart, lungs, or liver. Body immunity to disease peaks in adolescence but then steadily declines. Not that the number of acute infections increases in old age, for the opposite is true. Those over age sixty-five have fewer acute infections than those in the age seventeen to age forty-four group because they know more about how to guard against infection. However, when the older person does succumb to an acute infection, he is much less able to fight it and overcome it.

The Theory of Deliberate Biological Programming. This theory is based on the fact that most of our body cells (except brain neurons and cells of other vital organs) survive and rejuvenate by dividing and reconstructing as two healthy new cells. However, this normal human cell division—a basis of life—has a built-in limitation in that cells will only divide roughly fifty times and then die. Fifty cell divisions is the magic number and cannot seem to be increased in humans. This appears to be the determining factor of limiting normal life expectancy in humans to around seventy or seventy-five years.

Another example of deliberate biological programming is the fact that the human erythrocyte or nucleus of a red blood cell differs after cell division from its predecessor in having a smaller electrical charge. This smaller electrical charge reduces the efficiency of intercellular functions. With age and each succeeding generation of dividing cells, the electrical charge decreases even more, and the resulting cellular inefficiency is aging.

Theory of Accumulation of Deleterious Materials. This theory says that waste products and toxic substances collect in nondividing, nonrenewable cells. In aging our cells gradually overload with waste products that cannot be discharged.

Composite Theory. This theory is the most popular and says briefly that the fundamental aging process is the increased inefficiency of the organs whose cells are nondividing. In summary, aging is a normal and acceptable part of living.

We start aging after age twenty-five, but age twenty-five is not "over the hill." Learn to go right on living while you are aging. Don't be surprised when at age eighty-nine your mind is as clear as a bell; that is not unusual. That is normal. And at age eighty-nine, you are not "over the hill yet." You are on top of the hill, and that is the way it should be.

Reversible Longevity Factors	Years
Country vs. city dwelling	+5
Married vs. single, widowed, or divorced	+5
Overweight by 25%	−3.6
by 35%	−4.3
by 45%	−6.6
by 55%	−11.4
by 65%	−15.1
or, an average effect of 1% overweight	−0.17
Smoking—1 package cigarettes per day	−7 years
2 packages cigarettes per day	−12 years

Irreversible or Permanent Longevity Factors	Years
Females vs. males	+3 years
Mother lived to age 90	+3
age 80	+1.5
age 60	−0.7
Father lived to age 90	+4.4
age 80	+2.2
age 60	−1.1
Varicose veins	−0.2
Epilepsy	−20.0
Tuberculosis	−1.8
Trace of albumin in urine	−5.0
Moderate albumin in urine	−13.5

Ten Best Survivor Factors, By Rank of Importance

1. Most important factor - nonsmoker.
2. Having fewer illnesses, age forty to forty-nine.
3. Less worried (stressed).
4. Amount of smoking, if a smoker.
5. Better health, age forty to forty-nine.
6. Looked younger than age up to age forty.
7. Fewer illnesses, age thirty to thirty-nine.
8. More off-the-job physical activity, age forty to forty-nine.
9. Having a younger wife.
10. Conserved energy, slower pace, exhausted infrequently.

Other Longevity Factors

1. Being born when your mother was young (in her twenties).
2. Being a late maturer. (Were you the last person in your gang to reach puberty? Congratulations, you will probably live longer than the others.)
3. Living in a cold climate and getting out of doors regularly.
4. Staying out of the sun or wearing a hat.

The Longevity Commandments

Commandment Number 1: Be Positive and Hopeful About Your Future

To be positive and hopeful, you must come to good terms with the original Ten Commandments that were given to Moses and which Jesus summarized when He said, "Love the Lord your God" with everything that you are, and "love your neighbour" as much as you love yourself (Matt. 22:37-40).

Love the Lord your God. Find a meaningful life purpose which acknowledges God as Creator, Father, and Friend. Be positive in your life view as you discover just how good your life can be with God as your partner.

Enjoy your fellow humans. Find a meaningful life purpose which leads to a cooperative relationship with your neighbors.

Be hopeful, be constructive, and center your life's effort in an ongoing series of noble adventurous projects that are worthy of the investment of a human life. As an example of a noble adventure, has there ever been, in all of human history, a more exciting project than Bold Mission Thrust?

Commandment Number 2: Be Active, Physically and Mentally

The enemy is not age but inactivity. Inactivity knocks years off your life, but physical and mental activities rejuvenate and revitalize.

Don't be sedentary; don't vegetate; be a doer. Get moving. Vigorous physical exercise is a life preserver. The natural exercises of sitting, standing, walking, trotting, and running add months, years, even decades, to our lives and make us feel very much better.

Sitting and standing, when possible, are excellent exercises for the final years. Slower walking and standing are ideal exercises for the seventies and eighties. Brisk walking is nature's preferred exercise for the fifties and sixties, and a daily thirty minutes of brisk walking is all the exercise you need to keep you at your physical best. Trotting and running, in moderation, are acceptable exercises for the forties. Consult your physician, and get moving.

Use it or lose it. If you don't use your heart, lungs, muscles, intelligence, or reason, then be prepared for all of these things to wither or weaken decades ahead of time. If you are already withering, then get active again and watch yourself rejuvenate.

Commandment Number 3: Break Bad Habits

Bad habits knock *decades* off your life. It is never too late to break bad habits. What are these time robbers?

1. Smoking. One pack a day costs you seven years off your life; two packs a day costs you twelve years off your life. But if you quit by age fifty or sooner, your life expectancy gradually increases to the same level as those who have never smoked. Also, cut down on the amount smoked, as one-half pack per day is much less damaging than one pack per day, etc.

2. Alcohol abuse and drug abuse.

3. Physical inactivity.

4. Marijuana use. This enemy will soon be public enemy number one if its use continues to increase. Marijuana causes permanent damage to the reproductive organs of both males and females, damages the limbic system of the brain and the hypothalmus (involved in appropriate emotional expression) and robs us of energy and willpower to resist temptations.

5. Reckless driving. If you want to die a violent death in your youth or be maimed for life, reckless driving is still the best way.

6. Televisionitis.

7. Overweight.
8. Poor sleep habits.
9. Frequent excessive exhaustion.

Commandment Number 4: Prevent Disease by Fighting Its Causes

Ill health speeds up the aging process by as much as 2000 percent. This means that a person suffering for one year from a major illness can age up to twenty years in that one year. Ill health is the major catalyst for rapid aging.

Prevent ill health and rapid aging by working to eliminate the following disease causes:

1. Smoking.
2. Alcohol abuse and drug abuse.
3. Poor diet, especially resulting in obesity.
4. Inadequate work and exercise.
5. Worry and hypertension.
6. Inadequate rest and relaxation.
7. Extremes of blood pressure, especially systolic.
8. Radiation (stay out of the sun, or wear a hat).
9. Frequent excessive exhaustion physically and mentally.

Commandment Number 5: Eat Properly

Eat sensibly; eat with moderation. Enjoy a wide variety of foods, but restrict triglycerides (fried foods, fatty meats, gravies, pastries); restrict cholesterols (egg yolks, liver, butter, cream); restrict caffeine; and restrict calories. Why restrict calories? Because moderate body weight is strongly associated with longer life. Stay slim but not thin.

Be cautious of all diets, and judge a diet by the following standards:

(a) A good diet does not promise too rapid weight loss.
(b) A good diet does not emphasize only one food or one class of foods.
(c) A good diet permanently changes basic eating habits.
(d) A good diet includes emphasis on physical activity.

(e) A good diet is a balanced diet and should recommend roughly 30 percent fat, 50 percent carbohydrates, and 20 percent proteins. This thirty-fifty-twenty calorie ratio avoids the high fat, high carbohydrate diet that contributes to arteriosclerosis, atherosclerosis, coronary disease, and hypertension.

The ideal diet of long-lived populations over the centuries has been low calorie, simple, low in fats and meat, high in fruit and vegetables, and with no alcohol or nicotine (or very small amounts).

Energy maintenance requirements reduce as we get older, but older persons are advised to eat more times each day, though sparingly. After age seventy, many older persons are more comfortable when they have five or six nutritious snack meals daily and one small meal at supper.

If you are 20 percent or more overweight, consult your physician and therapeutic dietitian.

Commandment Number 6: Work

If you want a longer life, keep working. The life-style for longevity is work, not retirement. In long-lived populations each person has a task and is expected to work at something as long as he lives, with a reduction in the length of the workday as age advances. Avoid the rocking-chair philosophy. Physical working capacity declines with age, but it is not an excuse to stop working. Do what you can do. Don't foolishly overdo it.

Mental working capacity declines only slowly and moderately. Older persons know more in total and are more self-controlled; therefore, they can do considerable mental work even at a great age. Keep your mind working in the service of all your ideals and values, including family, faith, business, profession, and interests.

To work means to produce. So, produce. Do housework, yard work, service club work, church work, woodwork, metal work, baking, sewing, driving, writing, counseling, helping, talking, etc.

Commandment Number 7: Exercise Whenever Necessary

Exercise is only of value if you are not doing enough physical and mental work to stimulate and energize your whole body and mind regularly. Work is preferable to exercise, but if you are not doing enough work, then exercise. Exercise is the deliberate stimulation and use of muscles, limbs, heart, lungs, memory, reason, logic, thinking etc., just for the enjoyment of the activity because we know these parts of the body and mind need regular vigorous activity for their maintenance and rejuvenation.

Many persons do not need to exercise at all in the second half of life because the work they do is enough to keep them in top form. But exercise is important for those who don't work enough.

(a) Exercise your body:
—after age 90—sitting, standing, and gentle walking.
—after 70 and 80—sitting, standing, and walking.
—after 50 and 60—sitting, standing, and brisk walks.
—after 40—sitting, standing, brisk walks, and easy trotting.
—any age—gentle stretching, bending, reaching, twisting, and pushing.

(b) Exercise your mind:
—any age—fifteen minutes daily of memory exercises keep our memory in top shape; but with no memory work or memory exercise, our memory slips badly.
—one hour per day of thinking, reading, and problem solving keeps all minds in good form.

Commandment Number 8: Rest as Required

Have adequate regular rest and sleep, or you may put yourself in grave danger of both physical and mental collapse. Physical and mental exhaustion can start serious, negative biochemical chain reactions in the second half of life in which strong, competent, honorable individuals become confused, disordered, and ineffective. Do *not* overload your schedule. Overload is occasionally unavoidable, but it must be infrequent. Remember that your body and brain cannot function well on the amount of sleep and rest with which you were able to manage in your youth.

Severe stress is exhausting. Severe stress requires us to have extra sleep and extra rest, and yet severe stress works against sleep. If this is a serious problem for you, and if your sleep is inadequate and unsatisfactory, it may be essential for you to consult your physician for a tranquilizer or sleeping aid. The abuse of tranquilizers and sleep aids by millions of people is *not* a reason to avoid tranquilizers if they are definitely needed. Many major depressions and significant mental confusions could have been avoided if adequate sleep and rest had been obtained in time.

Rest is not an option: it is mandatory. Rest is a critical longevity commandment.

Commandment Number 9: Relax in Two Ways: by Reducing Anxiety and by Reducing Too Much Tension

First, reduce anxiety. Any activity whatever reduces anxiety, but two anxiety reducers are better than the others:

A. Talking about probable causes of our anxiety and taking the necessary action. The necessary action is always along the line of promoting our survival, ideals, and aspirations, and it usually concerns purpose, meaning, safety, security, health, and proper attitude toward self, friendships, family, employment, and faith.

B. Talk about the anxiety-emotions, which are fear (the dominant anxiety emotion), sorrow, anger, and guilt. Talking about fear is the golden key to anxiety reduction. Express your fear in relevant ways to appropriate persons, and your emotional expression will calm you and will help you to think straight about long-term solutions to problems. *Second, reduce muscle tension* by moderate exercise and gentle stretching. Moderate exercise relaxes, but heavy exercise increases tension.

Gentle stretching removes muscle tension. An excellent natural stretch is yawning. Other good gentle stretchers are:

1. Slow neck rolls and bends.
2. Gentle back rolls and bends.
3. Waist rolls and twists.
4. Reaching as high as possible, first with one arm and then the other.

Relax by lying down for seven minutes after a meal. Relax by going for a walk, playing a game of cards, watching the TV news, or sitting and sipping a refreshing drink.

Relax in a way that is good for you.

Moses Said It Straight

The new nation, fresh from Egypt, was waiting in the desert wilderness to receive its constitution and covenant. When the covenant arrived, through Moses, it spelled out clearly the spiritual basis of a longer, better life—namely, love and respect for God and obedience to His statutes and laws. Moses did not require many words to drive home the heart of the message:

"You shall be careful to do as the Lord your God has commanded you; do not turn from it to right or to left. You must conform to all the Lord your God commands you, *if you should live and prosper and remain long* in the land you are to occupy. These are the commandments, statutes, and laws which the Lord your God commanded me to teach you to observe . . . so that you may fear the Lord your God . . . and *so that you may live long. . . .* If you listen, O Israel, and are careful to observe them, *you will prosper and increase greatly* as the Lord the God of your fathers promised you.

"Hear, O Israel, the Lord is our God, one Lord, and you must love the Lord your God with all your heart and soul and strength" (Deut. 5:32 to 6:5, author's italics).

4

Old Brains Are Better!

Destroying the Myth of the Twilight Years

In the years from 1935 to 1965 there was an unfounded myth in general acceptance that older persons exist in the twilight zone of life. This twilight of the mind was described as a general mental state in which older persons can only think slowly and illogically, and their memory and problem-solving skills have slipped to an ineffective level. The mind was supposedly in a twilight zone: not the darkness of night and death nor the brightness and clarity of day, but a period of shadows, fuzziness, confusion, and rapidly fading mental skills. This false myth of the twilight years misled the elderly themselves and caused them to be gloomy about the prospect of their final years. The myth also fostered the culture of youth and caused society to look with suspicion on its wisest citizens.

The myth has been destroyed by more adequate scientific research, and we now have proof that there is no overall decline in intelligence scores, at least among healthy aged persons up to age seventy-five and beyond. In fact, elderly persons "know" more, are wiser, and usually have minds that are as clear as a bell throughout the life span. But it is taking a lot of sharing of the new set of facts to reverse the floodtide of emphasis on youth, so the elderly can enjoy those honors that are rightfully theirs because of their vast store of knowledge and wisdom and their greater experience in problem solving. The myth has been destroyed, but the facts of intelligence and aging are here set forth again in the hope of helping bury this disgusting myth once and for all.

Many Old Brains Are Better

What are the facts about old persons and their old brains? Four facts have been well established.

First, those with an intelligence that was high in their youth—high means at the ninety-fifth percentile or higher—actually go on increasing their level of mental skills decade after decade to age seventy-five and beyond. These very bright older persons are the premium citizens of our society. There is no younger group of citizens who are their equal; and whether they are presidents, pastors, poets, or prime ministers, they handle their tasks with judgment and skill, and their names and accomplishments are legion. They are the strongest argument that old brains are better.

Second, those in excellent physical health and living in the community are another group of our brightest citizens, and they show no decline in intelligence before age seventy-five. They are living proof that it is not age that is correlated with decline in intelligence, but ill health that slows down old brains.

Third, those in life roles that provide regular practice of mental skills do not decline in intelligence before age seventy-five. Use your mental skills or lose them! Those that are mentally inactive do decline, but the mentally active elderly are excellent thinkers, learners, and problem solvers throughout the life span. The more active the better, short of exhaustion and fatigue.

Fourth, the highly educated healthy elderly also show no deterioration in mental skills before age seventy-five. Education and the habit of study and learning are guarantees of mental excellence in old age, when accompanied by good health.

These four categories of bright and persevering older persons do not constitute a majority, but they are an increasing minority as more and more older persons pursue an active and healthy life-style. More and more old brains will be better due to this pursuit of an active healthy life-style in the second half of life.

Many Old Brains Are Slower—Why?

Some older persons do experience rapid major declines in intelligence. What are the reasons for this? Are there corrective actions that can be taken by older persons which can lead to recovery of their learning ability, memory, and problem-solving skills? The rapid major declines in intelligence in older persons are usually related to certain specific factors. Without becoming too technical, these factors are described as follows:

1. A pair of researchers, Eisdorfer and Service, have studied the intelligence of the elderly. These researchers indicate that one group of the slower elderly—those who were slower to begin with —do decline with age. In fact, those with initial lower IQs are declining in mental ability in most skills by age thirty! However, the reason is that they do not make regular use of their meager mental skills, causing decline from lack of use.

It is encouraging that others have observed another side to this problem, namely, that those slower persons with diverse intense interests in sports, music, and social activities who pursue an active, healthy life-style decline more slowly or do not decline at all. George, the ice maker, never could learn in school, but played hockey, football, and baseball as a child and then as a teenager. His passion was sports of all kinds, and this led to employment as a young adult in a sports arena complex in his small northern hometown. The pay was poor, but the job was right for George, and he was so stimulated by this employment combination of janitor and sports that he kept his slow brain at its maximum functioning level throughout his life span. Even after retirement, George was a regular volunteer, taking tickets at the games and helping in other ways.

2. Other researchers, Botwinick and Berrin, report that high blood pressure and cardiovascular problems produce major drops in IQ at any age, but especially among the elderly. On the encouraging side, effective treatment of these problems by medicine

and/or changes in life-style and attitude results in dramatic recovery of intelligence.

3. Spieth has studied hypertension and its effect on intelligence, and reports that untreated hypertension reduces mental ability at any age, especially reduction in problem-solving ability. Again, medical treatment and change of life-style leads to recovery of this mental ability.

4. *Any* serious health problems produce intellectual deterioration, but this loss is usually reversible with medical recovery and resumption of regular activation of mental skills.

5. Those elderly with "average" mental ability show a rise or maintenance of their verbal skills and general knowledge in old age, but they show a measurable loss of mental ability in tests involving pressure of time and/or eye-hand perceptual integration.

Why do some psychological functions decline with age while some rise or are maintained? Why is there this classic picture of loss of nonverbal performance skills in the elderly when speed is required, and there is limited time for completion? Researchers seem to agree that this means that older persons are just as intelligent, but they perform less well because:

(a) Older persons are much more concerned about accuracy than speed, so they are penalized by loss of points because they study instructions more carefully and are slower to begin. However, if the time limit is removed, they do as well as or better than younger persons in these difficult nonverbal performance tests.

(b) Older persons have more problems with vision and hand steadiness.

(c) Older persons are more aware of their surroundings and can be distracted by extraneous sounds and movements, thus increasing the time required to finish a task.

(d) There is a *decline in use* of these nonverbal skills, so there is a resulting *decline in ability,* but a subsequent *increase in use* results in an *increase in ability* which restores ability very close to its level of peak performance. If those who have become slower had continued to make regular use of nonverbal skills, there would not have been significant decline in ability.

The Two Conclusions About Old Brains

What, then, are the two unmistakable conclusions about intelligence in the second half of life, and what strategies for living do these conclusions imply?

First, the twilight zone is an unfortunate error in the annals of modern psychology. Contrary to this view, old age does not imply feeblemindedness. In fact, many old brains are getting better year by year, while many other old brains are maintaining their high level of mental function. Think about it: Who is the sharpest, wisest mind in all of your acquaintance? Probably that person is a man or woman in his or her seventies or eighties, whose mind is as clear as a bell, whose knowledge is greater now than ever before, and whose insight and judgment are markedly superior because of all the years spent in the pursuit of knowledge and wisdom.

In support of this optimistic view of intelligence in old age, the Duke Studies on Human Aging were unable to find any demonstrable decline in intellectual function in a group of subjects age sixty to ninety-four, over a four-year period, while those age sixty to seventy-nine showed minor but not striking declines over a ten-year period, regardless of consideration of regular practice or health. Also, in support of hope for old brains, the Age Center of New England studied eighty-six male and female subjects between the ages of sixty-four and ninety, and then retested these subjects four years later. On retest 51 percent of these subjects declined in IQ scores, whereas 49 percent actually increased, making it clear that old brains hold up very well indeed with the passing of time.

Second, the other unmistakable conclusion concerning intelligence and aging is: A smaller number of old brains do decline because of health reasons (not because of age), while a larger minority of old brains decline because of lack of regular active use of mental skills. Let us make two observations about these major causes of intellectual decline.

1. *Ill Health.* Even a slight reduction in optimum health results in a corresponding reduction in IQ scores. What is the usual cause of sudden very *rapid decline* in IQ after age sixty-five? The usual cause is a reduction in health. A striking conclusion of Human Aging I, a massive biological and behavioral study by the US National Institute of Mental Health, reads: "All mental abilities are correlated better to degree of health than to age" (p. 102).

2. *Lack of Regular Practice of Mental Skills.* Atchley summarizes the research on the importance of regular exercise of mental skills:

"Overall then, the picture is relatively positive for older people in terms of psychological functioning. The important factor in maintaining mental skills into old age seems to be an environment which allows the mental faculties to be constantly exercised" (p. 70).

So, once again, we see strong support for the "use it or lose it" view. As adults grow older, are less active, and slip into a sedentary life-style of spectatorship and leisure, the mind tends to be less stimulated and less active, and mental abilities wither away from disuse. But it need not be so if we pursue an active life-style.

Helping Old Brains Help Themselves

The goal ought always to be optimum mental function throughout the life span. This goal of mental excellence is achieved primarily by the successful pursuit of *good physical health* and *constant exercise of mental faculties.* In addition to good health and mental exercise, there are also learning strategies that ought to be known by the elderly and workers with the elderly. These learning strategies are effective methods of training that help to improve the performance of older persons:

1. *Learning by Listening.* The elderly learn better by listening than by looking, and they learn even better when they can both listen and look. Lectures and sermons are better than books in helping the slower majority of elderly persons to learn new infor-

mation. Television is better still because it combines listening and looking.

2. *An Active Role in Learning.* The elderly learn best if they can have an active role in learning. There is no better learning situation for the elderly than a class discussion-lecture combination where the elderly can interrupt, ask questions, and share information. Great teachers of the elderly make sure that teaching is a two-way process of guided sharing and participation.

3. *Distractions and Interference.* Older persons are much more aware of their surroundings than are younger persons, and they are thus more easily distracted during the moment of learning. Distractions and interferences should be eliminated or reduced if possible, especially in the beginning phase of learning when the elderly are the most easily distracted. Quietness and fewer interruptions facilitate learning and problem solving among the elderly. Background noise is never helpful.

4. *Accuracy, Not Speed.* The elderly are much more concerned about accuracy than speed. They wish to be very sure that they understand the instructions. Give them time to study the instructions carefully. Remember that even when time is of the essence, the elderly are usually the last ones to begin a task because of their concern to understand the instructions correctly. However, they are often the first ones to be finished even though they started last. All of the elderly remember occasions in their youth when they misunderstood instructions and answered an exam question without first getting its proper meaning. From this they have learned that speed is less important than accuracy. Their motto is: First you get the instructions very clear in mind, and only then do you begin.

5. *Meaningful Learning.* The elderly have great difficulty in learning new material if they do not see the relevance and meaning of what is to be learned. They may need to be persuaded that the new material is useful before they can be persuaded to learn well. If the new material appears to them to be false information or nonsense, the elderly learn the material poorly. But just show

them that the learning will be beneficial, and they will then learn it well.

6. *Neutral and Supportive Instructions.* If you wish the elderly to do their best in learning, avoid threats and challenges, and present your request in a neutral or supportive manner. Say, "Mr. Brown, would you be interested to help me check out your vocabulary? It might be fun. How about it?" instead of "Mr. Brown, I have a vocabulary test for you, and you must try your best because it may affect your pension. It is terribly important that you do well on this test. Whatever happens, don't fail the test." The elderly cannot do their best when they are anxious or fearful of failure. Moderate emotional reactions, not anxiety and fear, are conducive to best efforts of learning, problem solving, and memory among the elderly.

7. *Slower Pace for Learning New Material.* The elderly have much more experience to bring to the learning of new material as a part of their process of integrating the new material into the large body of their present knowledge. The elderly must relate the new to the old, and this takes more time as the amount of knowledge increases. If new information is presented item by item in rapid succession, the elderly learn poorly. If the pace of presentation is slower, the elderly learn well.

8. *Organizing the Material to Be Learned.* Learning is enhanced when the elderly are reminded explicitly to use learning strategies. What are learning strategies? They are simply ways of organizing material for learning. "Memorize this list of places *alphabetically,* and it will then be much easier for you to learn the list."

9. *Mediational Techniques.* These techniques are aimed at *highlighting* the material to be learned. In highlighting we deliberately prefer the information that we judge to be most important. "Study this chapter, and pick out the *main ideas of* each subsection." "Study this city road map, and form a mental picture of the six most important streets or avenues." The elderly learn quickly by means of such techniques.

10. *Note Writing.* All age groups—elementary school children,

university students, and the elderly—benefit in learning from taking notes. But the elderly sometimes fail to bother to do the note writing, and they are then putting themselves at a disadvantage in learning.

This section of learning strategies is intended to encourage the elderly to go back to school if they so desire. The second half of life is a great time to resume one's education—to take courses, learn new skills, and follow old interests further. This section is important to refer back to after you enroll and pay your fees! Happy learning.

Does Your Memory Need a Tune-Up?

There are two basic types of memory:

1. Recall memory: "What was your telephone number when you lived on Seventeenth Avenue?"

2. Recognition memory: "Which one of these three numbers was your telephone number when you lived on Seventeenth Avenue?" 1._____2._____3._____

Recognition memory is not a problem for the healthy, active elderly. Only recall memory declines with age, and this decline begins at age twenty-five and continues at an even and steady rate on a "use-it-or-lose-it basis" (Atheson, 1972). Bright people do not lose their memories with age. People who exercise their memories tend to maintain them completely.

Memory can also be described in terms of the age of memories, and one system is classified as such: short-term memory—one second to two minutes old; long-term memory—two minutes to twenty minutes old; old memory—twenty minutes to forty-eight hours old; very old memories—forty-eight hours to length of life. Of these categories, only short-term memory decays with age, and the causes of decay of short-term memory are:

(a) Not taking long enough to consolidate new learning. (Consolidate means "practice and rehearse the new learning to be sure you know it");

(b) Not controlling interference and distraction.

What is the formula, then, for a memory tune-up?

Develop memory exercises for yourself that will increase or maintain *short-term recall memory.* Remember that adequate learning is the basis of memory improvement, so learn it properly in the first place, and you will not forget it. Practice memorizing number series—both telephone numbers and addresses, check numbers, social insurance numbers, birthday, birthplaces, the fifty states and capitals, etc. In memorizing say the material aloud, form a mental picture of it, and practice writing it down. These three aids to memory—saying, imaging, and writing—will help us to remember. For those memories which are weak from inactivity, fifteen minutes of memory practice daily for two weeks is all that is needed to complete the memory tune-up.

Learning in the Second Half of Life

Many women and men age forty-five are saying to themselves, "I've learned much more in the years from age forty to age forty-five than I learned in any other five-year period! Why did my amount of learning increase in the years after forty?" How many persons in the fifties and sixties are learning at a faster pace than before because their personal development and maturity permit it? What about those in their seventies and eighties who have a sparkle in their eye because of a course they are taking in history, philosophy, or church architecture? To them learning is fun. Learning means there is a future, and the future means hope.

A major segment of second-half living ought to be learning and education, but this learning should be less for the purpose of employment and more for the purpose of personal growth and the pleasure of expanding one's mind in exciting directions. When is the right time to take a course in finance, social issues, Chinese cooking, seventeenth-century European pipe organs, teaching adolescents, raising roses, or Africa Christian Missions? The right time is today or tomorrow or whenever you are able to enroll and take the course. Old brains enjoy the mental challenge that comes from learning and education.

5

Three Distinct Stages
of Adult Development

Introduction—Biology Guides Psychology

Adulthood represents all the years after puberty, so by definition it makes sense to view adulthood as one stage, not three
stages. If you are an adult, you are an adult—period, end of discus-
sion. Yet the research and evidence of both the biology and the
psychology of human adult development supports the view that
there are three distinct stages of adulthood, which are:

	age 20	age 40	age 60
Childhood and Adolescence	Early Adulthood First Stage	Middle Adulthood Second Stage	Later Adulthood Third Stage
	‹----A D U L T H O O D--›		

Although we have already briefly considered the biological,
health, and medical factors of the second half of life, especially as
these affect longevity and level of mental functions there is one
additional fact of biology to consider. This fact is our awareness
of changes in our physical strength—its growth, plateau, and
decline—and the effect of this awareness of growth and decline on
our outlook on life. It is the awareness of decline in physical

strength which precipitates the transitions from one adult stage to the next. Adult stages in relation to growth and decline of physical strength through the life span are:

Age 20		Age 40		Age 60	
period of progressive growth	*end of growth*	stability of growth	*beginning of decline*	period of regressing growth	*beginning of faster decline* *decline*
growth of strength		plateau of physical strength		decline of physical strength		faster decline
Childhood		**Early Adulthood**		**Middle Adulthood**		**Later Adulthood**

Childhood and Adolescence: We are aware that we are *increasing* in strength.

1. Early Adulthood: We are aware that we are *maintaining* our strength.

2. Middle Adulthood: We are aware that we are *declining* in strength, though it is a slow decline.

3. Later Adulthood: We are aware that our physical strength is in *faster decline.*

We see from these charts that human biology and human psychology are inextricably interwoven, and it is the gradual awakening of the awareness of biological decline that precipitates the mid-life crisis at age forty: "Help, I'm starting to go downhill; somebody stop me. What does it all mean? Where will it all end?" Again at age sixty, we sense the increasing rate of decline: "Hey, I'm going downhill faster and faster. What should I do?"

Carl Jung's Overview of the Life Span

An excellent introduction to the stages of adulthood is the view of the founder of adult developmental psychology, Swiss psychiatrist Carl G. Jung (1875—1961), who has left a profound mark on our understanding of adults. His views have influenced major researchers such as Daniel Levinson and the Yale study group.

Jung's Four Stages of Life

Birth	Age 20	Age 40	Age 60
14	35	transition 40	65
Childhood	Youth	(maturity)	Old age

These four important stages of life—childhood, youth, (maturity - Jung never named this one), and old age—are distinct and separate from each other and can be characterized clearly. Emotional problems arise when people deviate severely from the standards for these stages. For example, some older persons insist on acting as though they were still in their youth (world's oldest teenager syndrome?). Each stage has and ought to have psychic (emotional) problems peculiar to it, but these problems are opportunities in disguise. Why opportunities? Opportunities exist because working through these problems at the right time produces personality growth that carries the individual forward into the next stage of life.

Childhood, for Jung, extends from birth to the years just before puberty. For most children, the pressures and challenges of life are gentle and are an unimportant part of consciousness. Conflicts are resolved quickly in normal children, and these conflicts are not deep or severely distressing. There are no real demands of life because parents guide, provide, and protect. The normal child is naively curious, fascinated with his own world, and only dimly aware of the realities of life. If the child is faced with major difficulties, then the causes of these difficulties are rarely within the child's mind but are commonly due to one or more of:

1. Ill health.
2. Family problems.
3. Social problems.

Youth (the years from 14 to 35) includes puberty and stretches to the period of transition, which is in the late thirties. The demands of life begin to crowd in upon consciousness, and we begin to use our energies to meet these demands. At times it is the sexual impulse that brings to an end our childhood, as we look beyond family for friendship, partnership, and intimacy. Just as often it is a sense of weakness and inferiority that propels us toward education, training, and the hard work that leads to accomplishment and a sense of adequacy. What are the major emotional problems of this fourteen-to-thirty-five-age group? (a) rebellion against the requirement to be self-disciplined (preferring instead to indulge cravings for pleasure and power), and (b) rebellion against the requirement for self-sufficiency (preferring to live on means provided by someone else). Thus, disturbed youth wants to remain a child, to do little, to extend the privileges of childhood but have the freedom of adulthood. Problems of youth arise when we do not let go of childhood, especially when our consciousness consists of:

1. Exaggerated expectations.
2. Underestimation of difficulties.
3. Unjustified optimism.
4. A negative attitude.

Solutions for the problems of youth arise when youth succeed in resolving these same problems by:

1. Trimming expectations.
2. Estimating difficulties accurately.
3. Behaving in line with justified realism.
4. Achieving self-discipline.
5. Accepting the requirement to be self-sufficient.

Finally, Jung points out what many others have also observed, namely, it is strange but true that young people who have to struggle hard for their existence are usually spared many inner problems, while those for whom life was made very easy find it a difficult struggle to gain and keep a mature perspective.

The focus of youth is an attempt to reach out and try our hand at making a mark on our corner of life. We desire to extend ourselves and see what size of parcel of life we can seize, subdue, possess, and enjoy. Aggression and daring are acceptable in youth, provided we respect the rights of others. The primary self-evaluations of youth arise from our success in making our mark. Our youthful estimate of self is related to our success in the world in our main lines of endeavor: marriage, employment, and friendship. The measure of the person, from the point of view of youth, is not the inner person but the person in the world and the size of his success when compared to his peers. Comparison is the criterion: "Am I doing *as well as* . . .? As well as my brothers, sisters, or peers? How do I compare? How do I stack up against so-and-so?" It is all relative: "My relative success when compared to so-and-so. My bank account compared to so-and-so's bank account . . . my house . . . my car . . . my job . . . my wife . . . our children . . . compared to his, her, or theirs." "My intelligence . . . my potential for the future."

The period of transition (the years from 35 to 40) separates the periods of youth and maturity. In this five-year period (which may come several years early or late), a significant change takes place in the person. It is a psychological change, as the person becomes bored with the task of making one's mark on the world and begins to enjoy an inner search and attempt to increase self-knowledge.

As *maturity (the years from 40 to 65)* begins, there is a maturity of consciousness. In normal persons, this maturity is brought about by an awareness of a powerful inner process forcing the contraction of life, an awareness that we are beginning to shrink, decline, weaken, and contract. Our sphere of influence is crystallized and possibly receding. Maturity makes us more responsive to reality, and reality warns that we are beginning to decline in physical strength. We are no longer aggressively seeking out and overpowering; we are now slowing down. Our new era is an introspective one where the inner self is to be enriched. What will be of help to us in this introspective era? Jung answers that religion becomes helpful at this point because the very aim of religion is to transform human beings into new persons (bring them to the next stage of life) and to allow the old forms of life (in this case the ways of childhood and youth) to die. Religious faith then becomes the true school of the second half of life, enriching both maturity and old age by building a stronger inner self.

In these years of maturity, each person takes a new reading on self. He begins to devalue his worldly successes and conquests and looks for a whole new way to estimate his worth as a person. In his view, self-estimate emphasizes character, integrity, wisdom, and the universal values of justice, kindness, courage, and love. He becomes more concerned with evaluating life than making an impact upon it. Meaning is the goal, not pleasure and endless activity.

Old Age Begins at 65. Jung observes that old age is similar to childhood in that both periods have fewer conscious problems. The fascination with the world (which is youth) is over, and the fascination with the inner self (which is maturity) has tapered off also. What remains is a focus on wisdom and the proper functions of a wise man or woman.

What are the two proper functions of a wise person? First, we survey life from the perspective of experience, having lived much of it, to look back (retrospection) with acceptance on what has happened, without forever wishing it could have been different. This is an acceptance of the past as it was.

Second, we find opportunities to share this wisdom with any who want it. Old men and old women discover that there is rich meaning in old age as they share their wisdom. Otherwise, old age becomes a meaningless pitiful appendage to life's day, a lengthy dying, a mournful, useless withering away. Not to share one's wisdom means not to live fully. Sharing one's wisdom means embracing old age and living it for its true purpose.

Jung's overview of the life cycle emphasizes the psychological aspect—a person's attitudes, motivation, and expectations—in response to a body that is first growing, then holding its own, and then in decline throughout the second half of life. The four stages of life focus on four questions concerning self and the world:

1. Childhood: Who am I?
2. Youth (early adulthood): What mark shall I make on the world?

3. Maturity (middle adulthood): How can I enrich my inner life and clarify my purpose as a person?
4. Old age: What have I learned about life that is worth sharing with younger persons?

The answers that Jung gave to these questions are a good introduction to human adult growth and development. Others who followed Jung appreciated his perception and broad understanding of how the biological and psychological aspects blend together harmoniously in normal persons.

Similar Overviews in Graphic Form

Daniel Levinson et al

	17	22		40	45		60	65
childhood			early adult era		middle adult era		Late adult era	

Levinson's view is similar to Jung's view except that Jung's period of transition is moved five years ahead from age forty to forty-five, and two more transitions are added at age seventeen to twenty-two and age sixty to sixty-five. There is even a shorter age thirty transition. Levinson's helpful point to consider is: The stages of life do overlap, and these overlaps or transitions are full of change, redirection, stress, and opportunity to move forward in living. So make the best of the transitions.

Erik Erikson's Adult Stages

	20		40		65	
childhood		Early adulthood		Adulthood		Maturity

Life's unfolding brings a number of natural crises which must be resolved for life to be enjoyed. *Early adulthood* must focus on intimacy versus isolation, answering the question "Can I form a durable intimate attachment to a peer?" *Adulthood* focuses on generativity versus stagnation, answering the question "Shall I widen my circle of friendships, begin new activities, and help other people, or shall I stagnate?" *Maturity* (beginning at age 65) focuses on integrity versus despair, answering the question "Shall I accept and understand the role that death plays in the life cycle?"

Frenkel-Brunswik

	17	28	48	64
Living at Home	Preparation	Culmination	Descent	Retrospection

Culmination is the most fruitful period in professional and creative work. Descent contains negative dimensions such as ill health, loss of associates, death of relatives and friends. Retrospection is marked by more evident decline, life review, reminiscence, and a gradual acceptance and understanding of death. This large statistical study took place in Austria in the 1930s, but its view is confirmed by biologists as well as psychologists (Newgarten and Birren) that physical decline becomes self-evident and undeniable at age forty-eight. It also supports Levinson's view that there is an important transition at age twenty-eight to thirty.

J. E. Birren

	17	25	50	75
Childhood	Early Maturity	Maturity	Later Maturity	Old Age

The similarities of Birren and Frenkel-Brunswik are clear, both emphasizing an early period of preparation in the late teens and early twenties. Birren pushes old age ahead ten more years, to age seventy-five, possibly reflecting the longer life-expectancy of his more recent study.

José Ortega Y Gasset

	15	30	45	60
Childhood	Youth	Initiation	Dominance	Old Age

Five equal fifteen-year periods: Is life as neat as this? Initiation is an interesting concept, followed by dominance. Do we spend our thirties and early forties getting initiated to the real issues, acquiring our skills, correcting our basic direction to life a few degrees, or right before the heaviest responsibilities are placed on us in the late forties and the fifties? Very possibly so for many of us.

Common Themes of Havighurst's Developmental Tasks

COMMON THEME	AGE 18	YOUNG ADULTHOOD	AGE 29	MIDDLE ADULTHOOD	AGE 64	OLDER ADULTHOOD
Finding a spouse		Selecting a mate (or adjust to singlehood)				
Relating to spouse		Learning to live with spouse		Relating to one's spouse as a person		Adjusting to death of spouse
Parenting		Raising children		Helping one's teen-age children into adulthood		
Choosing place of residence		Managing a home				Establishing satisfactory living arrangements
Selecting occupation and income		Starting an occupation		Making an adequate income		Adjusting to retirement and reduced income
Relating to the community		Beginning to assume community responsibilities		Leading in the community		Continuing in community and social obligations
Enjoying social affiliations		Attaching to a congenial social group				Accepting identity with one's own age group
Maintaining health and physical strength				Adjusting to physical decline		Adjusting to decreasing health and physical strength
Relating to aging parents				Adjusting to aging parents		

Havighurst's Developmental Tasks of Adulthood

Another dimension of adulthood is the developmental tasks which need to be learned and improved in each of the stages of adulthood. Robert Havighurst has organized the years of adulthood, not around the psychological and emotional crises, which are the focus of Jung, Erikson and others, but around those basic living skills that are important in each adult stage. While the above charts are fresh in mind, it is instructive to see Havighurst's adult stages in graph form, and then discuss the corresponding developmental tasks.

	18		29		64	
Childhood		Young Adulthood		Middle Adulthood		Older Adulthood
		11 years		35 years		11 years average

Notice the lengthy period of middle adulthood—thirty-five years—and see the equal lengths of young and older adulthood. Notice how, once again, young adulthood, ages eighteen to twenty-nine, coincides with a similar age span in Frenkel-Brunswik, Birren, and Ortega. Nine common themes which interconnect the adult stages can be identified, though Havighurst does not identify them by theme as is done in the diagram on the previous page:

1. *Finding spouse.* This is a task which most commonly occurs in young adulthood, and it is the most difficult of all the developmental tasks. Why the most difficult? Hollywood romance, decaying social and moral values, and false priorities have developed (in many young adults) false ideals and conflicting expectations of marriage.

These false ideals such as "Beauty is skin deep," "Marriage must be perfect," "My rights are what counts," "True love is continual ecstasy" often lead to a wrong choice of spouse.

2. *Relating to spouse.* This theme is paramount in all three adult stages and is the most complicated of all the life skills because it involves intimate skills, emotional skills, interpersonal skills, social, financial, and home management skills. Deficits in any one of these skills can endanger the whole marital relationship.

3. *Parenting.* In young adulthood this skill involves starting a family and caring for small children; in middle adulthood it in-

volves completing the task of preparing the teenagers for adulthood. Parenting is almost as complicated as marriage because in addition to the parent-child relationship, parenting also involves teamwork and cooperation with spouse.

4. *Place of residence.* Typical residences of the adult part of the life span: first, single-family dwelling or apartment, then smaller dwelling for couple, then smaller residence for surviving spouse, then retirement center, then nursing home care.

5. *Occupation and income.* This is another lifelong concern, which changing technology, unemployment, and ill health can make more difficult. Also, our increased expectations ("I would die without my microwave and video") cause pressure for a continuing rise in income, along with pressure to keep up with the Joneses.

6. *Relating to the community.* Another lifelong concern and need to be a contributing member of society.

7. *Social affiliation.* Important in young adulthood but important in older adulthood as well.

8. *Health and physical strength.* Of increasing concern with increasing age.

9. *Relating to aging parents.* A primary concern in middle adulthood.

These nine categories of developmental tasks may or may not be exhaustive in scope, but they do represent central and critical life skills. Havighurst's challenge is: If you are weak in any of these critical areas of endeavor, do whatever you can to improve. Take courses, get counseling, think, make wise changes, break bad habits—do whatever is necessary to strengthen your weaker skills, because fulfillment in the adult stages depends on success in each of these main lines of endeavor.

The Ideal Adult of Scripture

The studies of Jung, Erikson, Levinson, and other social scientists are *descriptive* studies of human adulthood. These studies are in the scientific tradition, in which science limits its work to a description of adult behavior without making value judgment.

The Stages of Life

	Birth	Age 20	Age 40	Age 60
Stage	Childhood and Adolescence	Early Adulthood	Middle Adulthood	Older Adulthood
Bodily Function	Growth	Maintaining Physical Strength	Declining Physical Strength	Faster Decline in Physical Strength
Mind Functions	Fantasy	Physical and Mental Strength	Mental Strength	Wisdom
Energy Direction	Play	Play and Work	Work	Work, Rest, and Play
Sense of Responsibility	Beginning Responsibility	Growing Responsibility	Greatest Responsibility	Variable Responsibility
Relationships	Dependency	Intimacy	Comradeship	Friendship
Income	Poverty	Prosperity	Wealth	Variable Finances
Identity	Self	Marriage	Family	Family and Community and Self

What are forty-year-old males like? How are forty-year-olds similar to fifty-year-olds, and how are they different? These are the kinds of questions scientists ask. The scientist counts, measures, experiments, and in the end describes the traits, qualities, behavior, and processes of adulthood. We have looked briefly at some of the important researchers in adult developmental psychology, and any book on human adult development and the life span is enriched by considering the findings of science on this subject.

But Scripture goes much farther than a description of human adults. Scripture is prescriptive and focuses not so much on how life is, but rather on how human adult life experiences ought to be. What kind of person ought I to be? What should the second half of life become? What was God's purpose in creating the human race, and what did He have in mind for the second half of human life? What is the meaning of being a person? What moral values lead to a better second half of life? How can a person have a basic change of mind and life in order to adopt a higher standard of conduct? What are some dangers of life—pitfalls, temptations, and distractions—that can prevent a person from making the best of the second half of life? What attitudes and habits can stand blocking the way to joy and satisfaction in second-half living? What is the scriptural and Christian view of the ideal adult in the second half of life?

These questions are the major focus of the chapters ahead. Each chapter will outline the relevant scientific findings and will be followed by the related scriptural and Christian considerations about the will of God, the meaning of human life, and those attitudes, beliefs, and values that portray the ideal Christian adult.

The major topics of the chapters ahead are the six identifiable segments of the second half of life, which are:

1. Mid-Life Crisis—The Road to the Better Half.
2. The Productive Years—45 to 55.
3. The Happy Time—55 to 65.
4. Growing Older—65 and Up.
5. The Closing Years—A Study of Dependence on Others.
6. The Crowning Years—A Study of Dying.

Two extra chapters cover (1) attitude and outlook; (2) an overview of the second half of life.

Part II
The Life Span

6

Mid-Life Crisis—
The Road to the Better Half

The Best Advice a Counselor Can Ever Give

"Think this over for at least seven days before acting upon it. It may *not* apply to you directly."

We have only just finished the introduction of this book—that's right, five chapters of a broad and general introduction to the second half of life: the principles, the opportunities, and the pitfalls of all the years after thirty-five. This general type of information in these chapters can be applied immediately and directly by each reader, and it is useful to help a person get his bearings and make plans for the second half to be the better half of life.

But the six segments of the second half of life, which are covered in the next six chapters, contain very detailed and specific information, and this information must be interpreted by the reader before being applied. The reader's interpretation is essential to be certain that the information and advice is applicable. There is always the possibility that the information is *not* applicable because any given reader may be a few years advanced developmentally, or a reader may be lagging behind several years developmentally and is not yet ready for the ideas and changes that are being considered.

As an example, Gus came to puberty late and has always looked young for his age. At his present age of forty-one, Gus looks years younger. In fact, he is still absorbed in the functions and goals of young adulthood. With the specific information presented about male mid-life crisis—it usually commences in the late thirties or early forties—Gus could assume wrongly that he *must* fit into the norms and statistical averages presented, or else he is abnormal. But statistics, norms, and averages do not work like this, and it is still normal to be outside of the statistical averages presented. Why? This is because Gus's body and mind may be developing well and in proper sequence, except that Gus is very fortunate indeed to be aging and developing more slowly! If Gus is abnormal, oh to be abnormal and age slowly!

So the best advice a counselor can ever give is this: Think it over for seven days before acting upon it. It may not apply directly to you. You must interpret the information in the light of your life circumstances, which might reverse the counselor's recommendations if you had been able to tell the counselor those circumstances.

The balance of the material presented in this book will apply to most readers but will not apply to some. But it should not be difficult for you to use judgment and discretion in spotting those points and recommendations which do not apply to you for response that include your own unique circumstances.

Seeing Youth for What It Is—and Letting It Go

The stages of life have their own themes, and the theme of youth is: Find your own identity and become a person in your own right. During this stage, as the pressures of conformity and authority squeeze us, our small but growing inner self says, "Meet the demands of life your own way; don't get lost in the crowd; be an individual; express your uniqueness; dare to be different." Sinatra and eternal youth have a recurring theme: I'll do it my way. This emphasis on individuality is typical of youth and young adulthood. Young adults have to make their own mark and do it their way.

This busy struggle to be unique, to prove oneself, and to surpass others usually lasts for twenty years. Year after year, young adults run hard on their treadmill of achievement until, finally, the day dawns when they see the treadmill for what it is: a tough taskmaster. The struggle for achievement begins to lose its appeal. Comparison with one's peers becomes uninteresting. Suddenly "aging youth" is ready to revise and update its life goals and strategy, and mid-life crisis begins. This is the "noon" of life and time for a reassessment. Decision time has arrived when we begin to see the haste and the ego of youth. We desire to let go of this demanding ego and its ravenous need for strokes. We want to move forward to something better. We see youth for what it is, and we are eager to let it go.

Women at the Noon of Life

The menopause is not the female's mid-life crisis; however, the inescapable approach of the menopause—first twenty years away in the future, then ten years away, then only five years away—is a natural reminder to women that the sand in the hourglass of life keeps on running. The menstrual cycle—its phases and stages—is a clear mark of nature's time clock which many women use to rid themselves of the illusion of eternal youth. Rita prized her beauty in her twenties and was still pleased with what she saw as the thirties raced quickly by. Her graying was barely noticeable; her bulging was a battle but was under control; her sagging and wrinkles were minor after a daily morning facial redecorating. But menstrual changes and the inevitable approach of the menopause helped her to accept the end of young adulthood *without a crisis.*

A better way of understanding Rita's transition out of young adulthood was that she did have a crisis of aging and change which was prolonged and gradual over a number of years. "By age forty I had accepted my new role. I didn't know if I was middle-aged, or if there was another name for it, but I knew my youth was over. I wasn't an old adult, but I wasn't a young adult either. I remember how I changed my appraisal of my past—my youth; I was no longer appraising it by a comparison with my peers. I no longer tried to prove myself as lover, as parent, as housekeeper, or as cook. I no longer did things just to prove to myself and others that I could do them.

"When I was age forty-two, we had a large group over for supper and an evening. I got the other women to help; it was an easy evening. I didn't have to do it all myself as I would have had to do at age thirty-two. I enjoyed the evening and came through it without exhaustion. I didn't care what the group were thinking about my cooking, but I did care what I thought of myself as a person. I knew my priorities had changed a lot in the intervening years. Later, when my menopause arrived, I was ready to make the best of it—with anxiety but without depression."

The majority of women, on the average, seem to be more successful than males in crossing the mid-life bridge.

Many women seem to have a mini mid-life crisis at age twenty-eight to twenty-nine, which helps them return later to a more moderate crisis in the middle or late thirties during which they resolve without hardship those inner conflicts that remain to be resolved.

A minority of women procrastinate. They refuse to face the inevitable. By becoming totally absorbed in parenting, marriage, career, or a combination of these, they manage to get older without admitting it, and then go into shock at the menopause, or they go into shock over the empty nest. For several years they are miserable, and usually make family and friends miserable too, until they come to new terms with the future, find new goals, or new responsibilities arise. Hazel was a devoted wife and excellent mother who had no time to look ahead as she chauffeured the children, managed the home with Herculean energy, and tried to be the best person she could be under such circumstances. As the children reached adulthood, and as the nest emptied, Hazel was desperate for several years until she began a new and exciting career.

Not all women have a mid-life crisis. Some are fortunate to have goals and projects which will last a lifetime, and these goals and projects carry them through the stages of life. Such women make changes one at a time, now dropping a responsibility, now picking up a new role, and they do not experience the crisis of identity and self-understanding that typically occur in the mid-life transition.

These women are the fortunate few, but those who experience a difficult crisis are fortunate too because the crisis forces them to face facts and make changes that they would otherwise refuse to make. The mid-life transition is not a negative; it is a bridge that must be crossed, even if the crossing is unsettling. Mid-life is an opportunity to take inventory and to set your rudder and sails in the direction of new priorities.

There Is No Male Menopause

There is no male menopause. The male mid-life crisis is one of the mind and emotions, not of the body and the hormones. A small percentage of males (1 or 2 percent) do experience some physical symptoms around age forty: tension, insomnia, and sweating. But these physical symptoms are a consequence of anxiety and depression and are not due to the natural physiology of aging. Because the anxiety associated with the male mid-life crisis sometimes results in secondary impotence (not having a physical or medical basis), some males are persuaded that the male mid-life crisis is menopausal and physical. However, there is no evidence to support this view.

Some of the confusion about whether or not there is a male menopause is due to a hormonal disorder called the male climacteric. This medically treatable disorder occurs in only 15 percent of males, and it is not a natural consequence of aging as is the menopause, but it is due to a shrinking and underfunction of the testicles. The climacteric commences many years after the mid-life crisis. Mid-life crisis begins usually at age forty while the climacteric occurs on average at age fifty-three, long after the mid-life crisis. The male mid-life crisis is, then, a natural psychological development to help us face the need to adjust and change to new opportunities ahead of us and should not be confused with female menopause or male climacteric.

Males at the Half-Time

The male ego: Is it more easily bruised? Does the male hurt more when he begins to grey, sag, bulge, and slow down? Is it more difficult for males to let go of their youth? The answer is probably yes. Levinson, the Yale researcher who studied males in their thirties and forties, says 80 percent of males find the mid-life passage to be "tumultuous." Carl Rogers, the dean of American counselors, describes in a striking manner his own thirty-seventh year as a time of many questions and few answers, conflicts and no solutions, anxiety and depression.

Why does the male hurt more at halfway? Males are more often dreamers who catch a vision, develop a goal, and then work so steadily to achieve that goal that there are few minutes for reflection and awareness of the passage of time. Then suddenly half-time is upon them, they are caught offguard, and the future is shockingly close. These dreamer-achiever males often make the world a better place to be, but their life-style is particularly rough on themselves when the second quarter ends and they imagine there is still plenty of time for more first-half touchdowns.

Other males are caught off guard at mid-life because their life-style of overeating, smoking, alcohol abuse, and lack of exercise is making them, by age thirty-five or forty, feel as if they are sixty. The premature death of friends and peers reminds them that their own death might be imminent.

Still other males find the mid-life crisis a surprise because business success, increasing social status, and newfound self-confidence distract their attention from the steady fading of their youthfulness. Harvey, age forty, happily married and enjoying the progress of his teenage children, relied on the stability of his marriage and family to ensure him of his continuing personal adequacy. His steady progress up the corporate ladder, to increasing responsibility and income, seemed to tell Harvey that he was not only maintaining his life but expanding it. Where could evidence come from, then, that youth was over and a new type of life was directly ahead of him, to which he must accommodate? A sudden corporate transfer to another city for him and his family and a mild but annoying and persistent back injury were enough to stop Harvey and get him thinking about his life. Soon all of the recurring themes of mid-life reappraisal were swarming through his mind demanding to be considered. What a coincidence that anxiety and fatigue and higher blood pressure suddenly made him feel less adequate sexually, and shortly after the feeling there followed the fact!

When is the male mid-life crisis? Opinions on this question vary. Carl Jung, writing in the 1920s and 1930s, considered mid-life transition to be the years from thirty-five to forty, and he did not distinguish male from female in terms of onset and termination. Levinson believes that male mid-life crisis ordinarily begins at age forty or forty-one and lasts five years, and this five-year period, age forty to forty-five, is very possibly the most common period for male mid-life transition.

What is the focus of the male mid-life crisis? Again the answers vary. Carl Jung considered the mid-life crisis to be extremely complex and multi-dimensional, involving psychological, moral, religious, and existential values. Levinson sees males in a crisis regarding four special areas:

1. Their loss of youth.
2. Their awareness of their own mortality and death.
3. Their masculinity.
4. Their individuality versus their connectedness to family and community.

All four of these areas are deserving of consideration in the pages ahead.

Mid-Life as the Beginning of the Better Half

"There is a tide in the affairs of men,
Which, taken at the flood, leads on to fortune."

Mid-life, with its bouts of depression, confusion, and anxiety, is not the most pleasant of times; but it is a vital and necessary opportunity for changes that will lead to personal growth and a better second half of life. The mid-lifer who grapples successfully with the great questions and comes up with satisfactory answers has set the stage for a thrilling second half. Mid-life is a negative experience only if we butt our head hopelessly against the brick wall, refusing to admit that youth is ending and conducting an unsuccessful search for answers to questions about self values and life itself. Mid-life ought to end up as a positive experience, a positive crisis, a life-enhancing self-evaluation, an appraisal, a good preparation for all the years ahead. The soul searching of the mid-life crisis should lead to wise decisions that have positive consequences in all the years of our future. A good mid-life crisis is a good way to start the second half of life.

Does the mid-life crisis ever get postponed for several years? Yes, mid-life crisis can be postponed by the untimely arrival of other crises: demotions, transfers to a strange city, loss of a spouse, ill health. This means that mid-life crisis will occur (or resume) after the other crises have been handled first.

The mid-life crisis asks important questions about self, values, and life itself. The crisis is triggered by an awareness of aging and the end of youth and points ahead to the inevitable approach of death. Seven questions summarize the focus of the mid-life crisis. Let us look at these seven mid-life questions, and let us look for guidelines about how to turn the mid-life crisis into an effective personal growth experience:

Question 1: Shall I cling desperately to youth as long as possible, or shall I let it go?

Howard, in his mid-life crisis, felt compelled to deny his age of thirty-eight. He wore only fashions that were in style for the seventeen- to nineteen-year age group. His hairstyle (after rinsing out the gray), his accessories, his walk, his talk—all conveyed the late adolescent/young adult image. "Life is youth, and youth is life," said Howard to himself, so he fraternized with very young adults in a desperate attempt to stop the march of time and the process of aging. But it couldn't work out, and Howard became depressed. The heart of his depression was *sorrow* over loss of youth and *fear* of the second half of life. Why fear of the second half of life? His parents were miserable and unhappy in their later years, and Howard could not imagine his own years after forty as potentially joyful. Only seeing the very real happiness of his colleagues who were in their late fifties enabled Howard to remove his fear of the second half of life. With this fear removed, Howard was able to work successfully through the remaining mid-life questions.

All of us, like Howard, cling to youth for a while. After all, it is the known. But ahead of us is the unknown, which causes anxiety and fear. But the lesson is: When youth is over, let it go, and turn to embrace the new day and the next stage of life.

Question 2: What is my evaluation of the years of my youth?

This is a good question to ponder. As we look back in a life review that is in many ways typical of the life review of old age in our late sixties, we should form a view of the positive and negatives, enjoying the positive memories and learning from the negative memories. There is always a mixture of good and bad memories, but the importance of this evaluation of youth is a proper attitude about the "bad" memories. Our past mistakes are in some ways more relevant to the future than our past successes, because mistakes signal the need for change, correction, and improvement.

The mid-life crisis will be the beginning of a better second half if we use the mistakes of youth to readjust our direction and approach.

Question 3: Have I possibly missed a deeper meaning of life?

This is a question about human existence. Is there meaning and purpose for each person's life, and may this individual meaning point to a broader meaning and purpose of human life and the universe and existence itself? The proper time to begin to ask questions about the ultimate purpose of life is in adolescence and early adulthood, not the mid-life crisis. But mid-life is a good time to return to this question and study it again: with more knowledge, more experience, and a much better brain. Mid-lifers usually start with their youthful philosophy of life and religious beliefs and try to bring these up to date.

It has often been twenty years since mid-lifers last considered seriously what the ultimate meaning of life is. Their motivation this second time around is the awareness of the approach of their own death. It is strange but true that death itself (our own death off in the distance and/or the untimely deaths of peers) is the greatest motivator to consider life in its broadest meaning.

Question 4: Is there a special meaning and purpose for the second half of life?

Cover the bracketed answers on the right. Consider your own answers and compare them with the suggested answers in the brackets.

Youth is doing;	second half is	(THINKING).
Youth is learning;	second half is	(UNDERSTANDING).
Youth is knowledge;	second half is	(WISDOM).
Youth is struggle;	second half is	(REFLECTION).
Youth is haste;	second half is	(SLOWING DOWN).
		(SEEING THINGS MORE CLEARLY).
		(COMING TO OUR SENSES).
Youth is excitement;	second half is	(JOY).
Youth is ecstasy;	second half is	(JOY AND PEACE).
Youth is beginning;	second half is	(BUILDING AND COMPLETING).
Youth is grasping;	second half is	(LETTING GO).
Youth is a student;	second half is	(TEACHER).

Mid-life is a serious business, so take it seriously. Let go of the rules of youth, and find the new rules of the second half. There *is* a special meaning and purpose for the second half of life, but the special message is both general (the second half is about wisdom, reflection, sharing, and teaching) and specific (to correct some of the imbalance, shortsightedness, and false beliefs of the first half).

Question 5: What are my values, priorities, goals?

Values: moral principles, guides for conduct, and basis of relationships. Examples: Am I responsible for myself? Am I my brother's keeper? Should I love my neighbor? Does laziness matter? Is honesty important? Should I strive to be the best person I could be, or should I be the lowest person I can be without being caught? Is unthinking self-sacrifice the basis of good parenting? Is anger an acceptable response from a good person? Should my feelings run my life?

Priorities: Rank these from one to ten. One means a top priority; ten means low priority.

—Have fun
—Be a faithful spouse
—Make money
—Support the church
—Be a good employee
—Visit the sick
—Spectate at basketball NBA
—Be a good parent
—Try to be a completely good person
—Save money for a favorite interest.

Now look at your profile you have made. Ask yourself if you need to change some of those priorities in the years ahead!

Goals: What are some objectives I want to reach for? What do I want to be or to achieve? What do I think I will want to be doing at age fifty-five, age sixty-five, and up?

Question 6: What kind of person do I want to become?

This is the question that concerned persons ask regularly about themselves throughout the life span, not just at the mid-life crisis. If they ask this question regularly, then for them the mid-life crisis is much less of a crisis. The question is asked regularly because there is no final static answer. The answer can only come as an ongoing response to our conscience and the values we cherish. The goal is always to personify our highest ideals. We must struggle to shape our life in the image of these ideals. Mid-life sharpens our definition of these ideals, helping us to see more clearly what traits of character need to be chipped off the image because they are not consistent with our ideal. The process of becoming involves three parts:

1. Knowing where we are now as a person.
2. Knowing what kind of person we want to become, which is the focus of this question.
3. Devising a plan of intermediate steps which will take us from (1) where we are now to (2) what we want to become. This third part is the focus of the next question.

Question 7: How shall I become a better person?

Answer: Strengthen your *character*.

Character is a broad general term to describe all of a person's individual characteristics, such as beliefs, values, attitudes, goals, and habits.

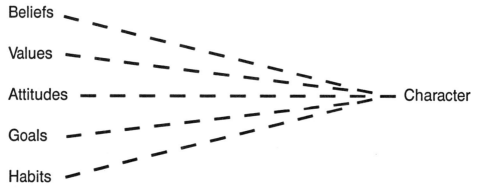

A character assessment analyzes the parts of our character to identify weaknesses and pinpoint changes we need to make. What are your character weaknesses?

You will not become a better person by worrying about it, but by planning specific changes of character and then carrying out your plans.

We are never too old to strengthen and improve our character, but it is hard work. The second half of life is a fine time for character overhaul and tune-up, and mid-life is the perfect time to focus on what character changes to make.

Decide to make changes. Perhaps your beliefs and values are in good shape, but attitude is a problem, or vice versa. Narrow down your areas of greatest need to change, and get started.

Comparison of Science and the Christian Ideal

Jung's Scientific View of the Life Span

14	35	40	65
Struggle of Youth	Crisis		Introspection of the second half

The Christian View of an Ideal Life Span

Birth	New Birth		The Years with Christ
	2 to 5 Years		The Struggle: Productive faith and witness
Before the birth of faith		The crisis of faith: a period of introspection. An analysis of the seven questions of life. An analysis of self, Christ, congregation, and community. Relating Christ to life's meaning.	After the crisis of faith comes the struggle of life, which lasts as long as health and strength allow.
This birth of faith comes by repentance, which opens all of the mind and character to major change.			First comes the crisis; then comes the struggle. The struggle is to live a life that is a witness to the fact of Christ in history.

Christ as the Crisis of New Life

The Christian does not find the current scientific views of the life span to be unacceptable, for they represent an accurate description of the average person's life. The duty of science is description: *tell it the way it is.* Jung, Levinson, and the rest are attempting to describe the life span.

The Christian view is prescriptive, not descriptive, and it therefore focuses on an ideal: *tell it the way it ought to be.* Science is the present reality, while the Christian view is the goal. It is not that there is a conflict here, but that there are two vantage points:

Science is the horizontal or factual viewpoint, while the Christian view is the ideal or vertical vantage point.

From the comparison (page 93) of the scientific and Christian views, look at the similarities and differences. Notice that the Christian views Christ as the great Crisis of human history, the source of light, the source of self, the source of values, and the source of meaning. Ideally the great crisis of life is the crisis of coming to Christian faith, and the sooner the crisis occurs in the life span, the better. The scientific view of the mid-life crisis is a fact: People do get serious about the meaning of life in the mid-life crisis when life is already half over.

However, this scientific fact is an unfortunate fact, and the better time to look for life's meaning is as soon as possible. Christ is the heart of the crisis, and the sooner a person comes to Christ, the more of his life is still available for the struggle. Notice how science and Christian faith place the struggle in opposite stages of life. Age forty is a good time for Crisis, if the seven questions of life have not been answered before age forty. However, thirty is better than age forty, and age twenty is better than age thirty as a time to face the fact of who is the Lord of life, and what the answers are to the great question of meaning and purpose. The sooner the great fact is faced squarely, the better the life.

The major process of Christian crisis is repentance, which is a radical commitment to changes of mind and values in the direction of Him who is the Crisis of history. Christ as Crisis represents the meaning of existence and the ultimate purpose and plan of every human life. But the Crisis of history becomes my personal crisis as I must choose Him or set Him aside. And if I choose Him, then I also choose the confrontation of His life and purpose and values with my own purpose and values, which is only resolved as I conform my inner self to Him.

My change of self resulting from the confrontation is repentance.

Struggle for the Christian is not a negative, but it is the essence of life itself. The struggle is the intention to live up to the ideal and to share the ideal and the Christ with other minds. In the

Christian view of the life span, first comes introspection (we think, study, and pray until we find the Christ of our crisis); then comes the struggle to remake our mind and life in the image of the ideal man of Scripture, especially by following Christ and serving Him.

But Christian realities always have some tarnish, especially those Christians who experience the Christ but fail to proceed beyond the infancy of faith and, therefore, respond to mid-life without the benefits of faith. For the Christian, mid-life ought to be less of a crisis and more of a review of basic ideals and a deepening of commitment to Christ and the virtue and wisdom that comes from His way.

A successful mid-life crisis paves the way to the years of middle age: forty-five to sixty-five. These coming years are the responsibility years of life, filled with productivity and satisfaction. In these years wisdom increases, and this wisdom frequently leads to joy.

7

The Productive Years— Ages 45 to 55

After the Mid-Life Storm

I remember a summer storm in my teen years on the family farm in western Canada. With a wagon and two horses, my dad, brother, and I went to get another load of hay, and the storm hit when we were only halfway home. We huddled under one side of the hayrack as the hail smacked the backs and rumps of the big black and gray horses, then left us and went on and destroyed all our standing grain crops. When we got back to the farmyard, there was lumber spread across the yard, broken glass, and one overturned shed. We walked around to check the damage, and then we set in to clean up and make repairs. The mid-life crisis is stormy too. The conflicts and confusions of mid-life sometimes lead to indiscretions, errors, and misunderstandings, but the subsiding storm within us gives time to survey the wreckage, if any, and we can start to make repairs wherever possible.

For some forty-fivers this is not a pleasant experience, but they look around at the main areas of their life; and, with better judgment and self-control, they repair, rebuild, re-create wherever they can, and set a stable and productive course of living. These are the productive years from forty-five to fifty-five. What is meant by productive? It is a relative term, of course, because youth was also productive in its own way as we acquired knowledge and skills; mid-life was also productive in a different way as our stresses and struggles with the seven questions yielded different answers. But the late forties and early fifties are productive in special ways:

1. We sense that we are at full adulthood at last with a new maturity and inner strength.

2. We learn faster than ever before, and we take on more and more social and career responsibility.

3. We let go of parenthood and adjust to the empty nest.

4. We survive the menopause and we are stronger than before; also, we revive the marital bond.

5. We revel in the magic of fifty and feel at age fifty-five that this truly is the better half of life.

Not that the productive years turn everyone into an optimist, for these middle-aged people have lived long enough that they refuse to wear rose-colored glasses. No, they are realists, managing as best they can in much less than perfect circumstances. But the storm of mid-life, in retrospect, is a positive experience that leaves them stronger in mind and will. They are not ready to give up, and they do sense, as they plan and work and build, that the best is yet to be.

Full Adulthood at Last

Sixteen-year-olds, imagining as they do that they have full knowledge and superior everything, "know" what it is to be grown up. Ten years later these same persons, now age twenty-six, are quite surprised that their elders do know a little, but they retain their exaggerated estimate of their own capability.

Another ten years later, these persons are now age thirty-six, and they are too busy to think about how great they are because they are running their fastest on the treadmill of youth getting everything done that they wish to do. But how different they are at age forty-six! At last they do have an understanding and knowledge of what it means to be a person, but they no longer have the need to crow about it. They understand now how very little they know compared to the total body of knowledge, so they share their knowledge with humility. The windbag of youth is deflated.

Age 16—full "knowledge" and superior everything.

Age 26—still confident but slightly subdued.

Age 36—too busy to think and even more subdued.

Age 46—very much wiser and quite humble about it.

Full adulthood means that we have a reasonably accurate assessment of our own strengths and weaknesses, that we can accept ourselves the way we are while at the same time working to become a stronger and better person. This achievement of full adulthood seems to take around forty-five years! Certainly some persons mature earlier, but the majority of men and women take four to five decades to really grow up. What is the first decade of full adulthood? Answer: age forty-five to age fifty-five. At last, men and women have that balanced sense of self, along with the calmness, concentration, persistence, and perspective that is the mature person. Forty-five to fifty-five = maturity = full adulthood.

In males this decade begins with the end of mid-life crisis. Because people are unique and different, the mid-life crisis does not usually end exactly at the forty-fifth year. In fact, it is possible for the mid-life crisis to end as early as the fortieth year, five years ahead of schedule, as it probably did in the life of Carl Jung. At the other extreme, there are some males who storm from age forty-five to age fifty with the calm after the storm only arriving around their fiftieth year. The length of the mid-life crisis may also vary in males. The average length is four to five years, but among those who have in their youth tried to face the questions of life squarely and introspectively, the crisis is often much shorter and less severe while the procrastinators and extroverts usually have a crisis that lasts five years or longer and has very stormy episodes. But long or short, mild or severe, the mid-life crisis leads to a calmer, satisfying, more productive period that is built on the answers that were found during the crisis. A significant minority of males do not experience a mid-life crisis as such, or they experience only a trivial crisis that is brief and inconsequential.

In females this productive decade straddles the menopause, which occurs usually in the late forties or early fifties. For the vast majority of women, the experience of the menopause is not a major distraction from the focus of this period because much of the psychological discomfort of the menopause has been experienced in anticipation of the menopause during the mid-life crisis. However, a small minority of women experience major episodic physical discomfort in the menopause, and for this small minority the menopause is a distraction.

Full adulthood in these productive years means we are moving ahead at full stride in the developmental tasks which are specific to this period as we outlined earlier by Havighurst. Moving ahead at full stride does not mean life is perfect; but whatever our circumstances, we are making the best of the situation. The common themes, which focus our endeavors, are relating to spouse or adjusting to single living, parenting our teens, and helping our grown children, maintaining our income, relating responsibly to the community, maintaining social affiliations, and relating to aging parents. In each of these categories we are doing what is possible, however little that may be, and we are doing it effectively. In addition, we are accepting the decline of our physical strength, which for most of us at this period is a very minimal decline.

A Definition of Maturity

Maturity of mind is the essence of this period. The humanists, existentialists, and others have all set forth their own definitions of what it means to be a mature person. In this analysis of the productive years, it is valuable to look at mature adults: what they are and what they are not.

Some Characteristics of a Mature Person

Relation to Self	Relation to Others
self-aware	self-controlled
realistic	moral
rational	involved
calm	compassionate
self-confident	assertive

focused
competent
persistent

having balance and
    perspective

Some Characteristics of Immaturity

Relation to Self	Relation to Others
ignorant of self	easily pressured by others
impractical	impulsive
controlled by emotions	passive or aggressive
unstable	detached or overcommitted
unsure or overconfident	self-centered
not goal directed	
unskilled and incompetent	
not persistent	
egotistical	

Mature persons have most or all of these qualities of maturity. Hopefully, where they are weak on one or more points, they are not glaringly weak, for one glaring weakness can nullify many good points. Mature persons are aware of weaknesses and exercise caution and care. They know they are not perfect and seek to prevent their weaknesses from bringing any harm to others.

Maturity is the key to productive living in this decade, but there are some persons who are very productive in some areas of their life while they contribute little or nothing in other areas. For example, John was a wealthy self-made man who owned and operated a very large dairy. His dairy ran perfectly because John gave all of his energy to it, but his family life was in ruins from neglect. John's brother Sig owned an adjoining dairy, but Sig neglected his dairy for family and sports. Sig had reason to be proud of his wife and sports-minded sons, but there was never money to paint the house because Sig's dairy always had its problems. Sig had always intended to do things better in his dairy, but for twenty-five years his intentions had not resulted in changes. Look at the chart on characteristics of a mature person. John had self-confidence, focus, persistence, reason, and competence in business. He lacked involvement in family, self-awareness, compassion, balance, and perspective. Can you itemize Sig's strengths and weaknesses?

Maturity has many dimensions, and it is surprising that there are examples of men and women who have major immaturities rooted deeply in their character. These men and women refuse to quit and gamely trudge forward toward their objectives, carrying these handicaps of immaturity with them, and they often make enormous contributions to family and community in spite of themselves. Billy was a Christian education director of a prospering congregation. He was very weak in administrative and organizational skills, and he had a bluntness that often bruised relationships. He shouldn't have been a success, but he was. He had such a clear vision of the value of Sunday School work that he could keep teachers at their work. The attendance and enrollment grew, and many benefited from Billy's vision. The Sunday School records were nonexistent, but the class members were doing well. Billy's contribution was very much on the positive side.

Sour at Fifty

There are brief spells of bitterness and despair at any stage of life, even in this late forties—early fifties decade. Deaths, accidents, injuries, misunderstandings, illness, employment difficulties, mismanagement of finances—any of these can bring a cloudy day or month or year. Not only one of these, but two or three calamities in rapid succession can take any one of us and bring us to our knees. Ancient Job was as ready as any person to cope with one or two personal disasters, but five disasters in a row? Job's calamities rolled over him like waves hitting the beach, one after another. Of course the important thing is not the number of calamities but the character of the person who is experiencing them. Why do some turn sour, and others remain sweet spirited? Maturity, attitude, and Christian faith—these three qualities certainly help to retain a sweetness and serenity in difficult times.

Still others, though they are a small minority, find this entire ten-year period to be a time of frustration and bitterness. Imagine such a contrast: the majority living exuberantly and finding fulfillment and contentment, and this minority unable to answer the seven questions. The minority cannot find a deeper meaning to their own individual existence; their values are contradictory, their priorities backwards. Those who enjoy these middle years cannot understand Gerald, who is always wanting more and is quite dissatisfied with what he has, seeming to have no idea of how very fortunate he is to have a wife like Ivy. Ivy listens to Gerald considerately as he rattles off many complaints that do not deserve serious consideration. Ivy is happy to be alive, after nursing her own mother who died at age forty. Ivy is already age fifty and considers all her years after forty as a gift of grace which her mother never enjoyed. Gerald is into self-pity if even his NHL hockey team loses, and he is quite into criticism of the team management or the game linesmen. Sour at fifty, after his parents made his childhood too good to be true and after Ivy spent all her time of thirty years married to Gerald trying in every way to increase his happiness, Gerald showed no signs of coming to the realization that he was his own biggest problem. Poor Gerald—no one else ever had it so good. But Gerald didn't understand this.

Why do some have eyes but cannot see, and ears but cannot hear? Very often these are the sour ones at fifty, while the majority are striding forward.

Am I Carrying the World on My Shoulders?

The second half is definitely the better half of life for most men and women, and if you are not positive of this, then ask the forties-fifties group. They like their lives—but they do have one complaint. They sometimes feel as if they have all the responsibility for their families, their grown children, grandchildren, aging parents, community organizations, and employer, and there are not enough hours in the day to meet all of their commitments. It is sometimes called the generation squeeze because middle adults are sandwiched in between younger adults (who *still* depend on them in many ways) and older adults (who are *just starting* to depend on them in many ways).

Harriet and Bill have three children in their twenties—all married and all with children. Harriet says, "Bill, we can't afford to finance the kids even if they are unemployed or between jobs or in a bind because of overcommiting themselves." But Bill enjoys being able to help, even if it puts more pressure on Harriet and him. Harriet also baby-sits the grandchildren often—when she enjoys it and also when she doesn't enjoy it but can't seem to say no. Then their youngest child Sally and husband came home to live for two years with a newborn. There were a number of other lesser ways in which Harriet and Bill felt responsible to help their children, and these ways added up to a grand total that was more than Harriet and Bill had ever imagined would be the size of an ongoing commitment to one's grown children.

The whole question of responsibility is a unique problem for persons in this age bracket because their predictable successfulness causes others to call on them for help. No is the most beautiful word in the English language at any age of life, but it is especially beautiful and necessary for the forties-fifties group. The most difficult no is spoken to one's own children and grandchildren, as it conveys the message, *no*, definitely *no*. "Yes, I do care, but my choice is not to help you. It is time for you to do this for yourself: *Tuum est*—this time it is entirely up to you." The word *no* in this instance is a responsible reply, while the word *yes* and the actions of helping would be irresponsible and hurtful to others in the long run.

Aging parents are another segment of the generation squeeze, and they add to the feeling of carrying the world on our shoulders. Aging parents may need help in a number of areas: finances, transportation (trips to the doctors, helping to move to a new residence or relocate, arranging to move to senior citizen's housing, or moving to a personal care home), visits (they may need to live close by and have us drop in on them once a day), accommodation (few would choose to live with us, but this is sometimes a practical arrangement), grooming (bathing, hair care, and toenails). The list of needs may be short in some cases, but in other cases it is a very long list of needs.

Employers also lean on those who are in the productive years. Middle management—doesn't it keep industry rolling? The very top executives look after policy matters and planning, while the actual operation of the whole enterprise depends on the group who are one level lower and one decade younger, namely the forties-fifties group. If something goes wrong in the business operation, call middle management. It can be a twelve-hour-a-day job, six days a week. No wonder this age group feels it is carrying the world on its shoulders! Add to this community, social, and congregational responsibilities, and the forties-fifties group is certainly doing more than its share.

It is at this time that many executives escape to the three martini luncheon, which only leads to more problems at home and work. Can anyone fault the businessman who escapes for a game of golf, tennis, or racketball: tension relievers which might ward off ulcers or, worse, a heart attack.

Breaking the Parenting Habit

During this decade—age 45 to 55—many parents do learn to let go of the responsibility for their children and grandchildren. This is a most difficult task because our instincts have to be denied, and thirty-year habits have to be broken. Harriet has to fight her instincts as she looks at this darling nine-week-old baby girl. Many voices inside her say, "Go ahead and have her for the weekend, so the kids can have a break." But these instinctive voices need to be opposed by reason and common sense which say, "I want to have this darling for the weekend, and I want to give the kids a rest, but I am building the second half of my life. Do I want to have my grandchildren as a *major* part of my time and energy or as an *occasional* part of my time and energy?"

Most parents decide to enjoy their grandchildren as an occasional part of their time and energy, and it is then their responsibility to define very specifically how often and in what ways they can be involved and on what terms. Some parents decide to have family as a major focus of their second half of life, and they would be unhappy with it any other way. It is quite a difference, and each person must make his choice. The *majority,* who opt for less responsibility toward family, find it difficult to break the parenting habit, and they sometimes find themselves helping children and grandchildren before they realize they are doing so. Habits are not easy to break.

Some effective ways to break or reduce the parenting habit are:

A. Tell your grown children you are thinking about your ongoing parental responsibilities and that you wish to reduce these commitments. This is the direct approach and should always be used first. Usually, they will be in hearty agreement. But when they are reticent about the withdrawal of your help, assure them that you do care for them but the responsibility is theirs, not yours, for their lives and the lives of their children.

B. Increase your commitments in those other areas of your life that conflict with parenthood, so you are simply not available at predictable times when calls for help usually come. If you are not available, you will not fall into the parenting trap.

C. If you were ever thinking about moving across town or upstate, maybe you should think some more about the possible move.

Everyone is different. Herb and Jean looked forward every year to their six-month trek to the sunny south. Letters and occasional phone calls are their only family link. They golf, swim, and tan. They come back for the summer and are parents, friends, etc., on a six-month basis.

Bob and Claire spend four to six weeks every winter traveling. For Claire it is about three weeks too long. She misses her family, her home, and her organized life. They can afford to be snowbirds annually, but she is not ready or desirous of splitting her life for the sake of the run.

Who is right? Who is more selfish? Neither. What is right for one couple is not right for another couple.

Enjoying the Empty Nest

The empty nest occurs when the last child departs from the family residence. The empty nest syndrome is the painful emptiness in the family-centered mother, who must make adjustments in expanding her interests outside the home in order to fill her emptiness. However, this syndrome is experienced only by a minority of women, while the majority find that the empty nest is an experience to be enjoyed. Recent research finds empty nest women to be more contented, more open emotionally, and less self-pitying (Campbell, 1975). Parents who describe their empty nest experience tend to report that it was more positive than negative (Hagestad, 1980). Only if parents or the child leaving showed some maladjustment did the empty nest have a strong anxiety component to it. Those in the forty-five—fifty-five group report high levels of life-satisfaction when the empty nest occurs (Glen, 1975), possibly because these sons or daughters maintained a positive relationship to parents after departing. So parents ought not to anticipate with dread the departure of their last children from the family residence, as this usually is a step forward in better-half living. Only those mothers with restricted interests should take warning; the rest will find it a pleasant time indeed.

Reviving the Marital Bond

Marriage is still the preferred life-style of a large majority of adults, and in spite of Hollywood and the mass media, the institution of marriage is statistically sound. Two thirds of all marriages last a lifetime. Of those marriages that do break down, 75 percent of these people remarry within four years, and 80 percent of these remarriages last a lifetime! That's a great record when we understand first that the social stigma of divorce is greatly reduced, and second, that the attitude of the young is that they now simply refuse to endure a painful relationship for very long for the sake of pride, parents, friends, or reputation. Their parents may have toughed it through a difficult marriage, but they have less patience and tolerance because they do not see the point.

So marriage is doing well, all things considered, but it has its ups and downs, and several research studies show that even sound marriages provide less satisfaction in the late forties, especially among women. Not that the marriage is doomed, not at all—but the couple are both in such an upheaval of change within themselves that the marital relationship has difficulty in maintaining a pleasant adjustment. He is learning a new attitude and outlook toward self, society, and the future. So is she. And the sheer volume of changes makes it easy for them to get out of step. But mature minds can resolve very complicated problems that previously were unsolvable. Many couples look at the relationship carefully and, after time, talk, compromise, and patience, make a better marriage.

Several points are important:

(1) Havighurst says this is the time to appreciate the spouse as a person and to realize that the sexual part of the relationship takes on a broader and deeper meaning of caring, sharing, and appreciation.

(2) Females come through the late forties and early fifties with a toughness of character and an increased determination that is almost masculine. Many males come through this period with an increased tenderness, gentleness, and consideration that is almost feminine. Such a change in both partners results in the need for them to study roles and responsibilities in the marriage, and a new arrangement may improve the relationship. Usually, the outcome of this masculine-feminine change in both partners is a much more understanding and equitable relationship.

(3) Counseling is important in marriage at any time that it is needed, but at this stage of the marriage, counseling is even more important in order to protect the huge investment of many years. Don't take a risk; get the counseling if it is indicated.

The Menopause—Time to Make a Fresh Start

The physical discomforts of the menopause, including "hot flashes," headaches, nausea, dizziness, and heart palpitations, are serious for a small minority of women. The majority of menopausal women do not, however, find their experience to be a major physical discomfort. There is often anxiety, expressed in the statement "So far it has not been too difficult for me, but will it get much worse? I don't know. Will I be incapacitated for a time? What if it is worse at a very inopportune time? If what I have already experienced is the worst part, then I will look back on it as an easy time, but how bad will it get?" But for many women, the expectation is worse than the experience.

The psychological effect may also be quite negative in terms of brooding on physical symptoms and depression about the loss of capacity to bear children. Women also ask themselves questions about the effect of menopause on their sexual interest and capacity. But the menopause is usually a positive experience of personal growth, resulting in increased self-confidence, courage, and optimism. Postmenopausal women tend to be mentally stronger than ever. They enjoy their freedom, and the new horizons that they are considering often become major sources of satisfaction that were unknown to them in their premenopausal life.

Have I Graduated from the School of Hard Knocks?

Age twenty is an accomplishment, and we are looking forward to good things, but at ages thirty and forty we are unsure, looking forward and looking back, and wondering if we are over the hill. Frank was quite depressed at his thirtieth birthday party, especially when friends made him a celebration cake with *black* icing and black candles. The black cake was his view of the future, with gloom, clouds, weakness, darkness, and death. Was there life after thirty? Is growing old the living death after youth?

The Big Five-O with fifty candles on the cake is the first decade milestone that is once again full of hope for the future. To reach age fifty is an accomplishment. Congratulations! The basis of optimism at fifty is the sense that the different strands of life are coming together, flowing together, and blending together in a unity and oneness of purpose. Fifty-year-olds sense that they are at last getting it all together, and their inner self is becoming a meaningful whole. Inner conflicts are mostly settled, and there is a peacefulness that comes from having goals, priorities, and strategies which are consistent, realistic, and attainable. The second half of life is truly a time when we begin to make sense of what it is to be a person. Our efforts toward better living bear fruit, and the second half of life does gradually build in satisfactions and fulfillment.

Is this the graduation from the school of hard knocks? Yes, it is. What does it mean? It means we now know enough about ourselves and others that we can learn the lessons of living the easier way, not simply by getting hard knocks over the head. The fifty-year-old is glad for past mistakes because he feels he has learned from them, so he will not have to make the same mistakes again. Life is going to be smoother sailing ahead because we have graduated from the school of hard knocks, and we are now attending the school of "thinking first before we act, having our ego in control so that pride does not trip us, placing reason before feelings, and having realistic expectations of self and others."

In the school of hard knocks we were not listening to good advice (because we already knew everything), and we butted our head hopelessly against the mountain of granite. In the school of the second half of life we listen with humility—or we ought to—and the consequence is fewer heartbreaks, fewer disappointments, fewer losses and failures. We still have some lessons to learn by trial and error, so there are still some errors. But what a good thing that we remember the lessons of our mistakes, so we do not need to make the same mistakes twice.

8

The Happy Time— Ages 55 to 65

Happiness Is Never an Accident

"Believe me, my happiness didn't just happen. After forty, I started to catch on to the formula for happiness, and planned, and worked at it many years ahead. It is no surprise that fifty-five to sixty-five was so good because I had already been busy setting my life up for this special time. In fact, it would have been surprising if I was *not* happy. After all, life is not so complicated. Life can be figured out, and happiness can be the result of sound planning and strategy.

"Luck and chance—what do they have to do with it, unless occasionally the law of averages goes against you? But when a series of misfortunes occurs, isn't it often followed by good fortune, too, so that it has a way of evening itself out?

"We make our luck. We make our fortune, at least for the most part. So if things are tough, smarten up. See what changes you have to make. Don't blame it on bad luck."

Do you agree with these tough words from Bob? In his late seventies, he seemed to have a practical philosophy for pursuing happiness by not pursuing it. Listen to his punch line, "I don't mean that I am always trying to be happy or that happiness is my goal. My goal is: Be sensible, work hard, treat people right, be friendly, and don't be a big mouth. Then my happiness came as a reward or spin-off when I succeeded in doing these other things."

111

Happiness is never an accident. It is the reward for getting your life together.

Six Sources of Life Satisfaction

Fifty-five to sixty-five is the favorite decade of life—the best part of the better half. Older adults who look back on their life span to select a decade when they were happiest usually choose the late fifties and early sixties. This is the period that they recall as being the most enjoyable.

What are the main sources of life satisfaction? What do these sources mean, and how are they obtained? Let us look carefully at six major sources of life satisfaction and examine how and why these sources flow in abundance in this decade. As we look, let us keep in mind that these same six sources continue to be the basis of life satisfaction in all three remaining segments of the second half of life, which are, first, older adulthood, second, the closing years, and third, the crowning days.

Wisdom: Getting It All Together

It is quite an achievement to put a life together so that it has meaning and unity. This doesn't happen overnight, and more often than not it takes fifty years or longer. Those in their late fifties and early sixties feel that at last the separate strands of life—values, beliefs, attitudes, goals, and skills—are blending together. The separate strands are no longer separate but are weaving together to become one pattern, which is the person they want to be. There is a unity—a central purpose—which is usually the goal of "being the best person I can be under the circumstances, investing my life in the service of my highest values."

What is wisdom? Wisdom is the practical application of knowledge. Wisdom is the broad perspective that sees the forest *and* the trees. Wisdom gets it all together—the values, beliefs, and goals—so that persons manage their lives effectively, efficiently, and consistently.

The theme of the first half of life—all the years from birth to thirty-five—is action: "Let's do it." "Let's do it for all we are worth." "If it is a square peg that has to go into a round hole, then hit it harder. It has to go, so drive it."

The theme of the second half of life is wisdom. "Let's take our time at the beginning to see the opportunity in its full perspective. Let's come up with a good plan, make the preparation, and then, let's do it for all we are worth. Square pegs won't go into round holes, so let's redefine the task so we can make sense of it."

Wisdom is not only the theme of the second half of life; wisdom is also the purpose—the *raison d'etre*—the reason for existence— of the second half of life. This purpose of the second half of life is the acquiring of wisdom and the sharing of wisdom with others who do not have it.

Certainly those who are in their late fifties and early sixties ought to conduct their own lives wisely, and they usually do this. But the highest fulfillment of all the years after fifty-five comes not merely from managing your own life wisely but from sharing your wisdom with others who need it. It is the sharing of wisdom that brings joy, at least where the wisdom is recognized and appreciated. The wisest persons of all manage their own lives so that the sharing of their wisdom will be a primary focus of all the years after fifty-five. They see ahead to the time when they will be age sixty, age seventy, age eighty, and age ninety; then they determine that they will cultivate a reputation for wisdom, a reputation for a willingness to share their wisdom, and a reputation for friendliness and understanding. If they do this throughout the second half of life, persons who need their wisdom will be beating a pathway to their doors to enjoy the benefit of their wisdom.

This is exactly the formula many have followed who are finding such joy in all their later years: They live a life of sharing their wisdom and expertise. They started this in their forties and fifties on a smaller scale because in those years, their wisdom was on a smaller scale. Now in their sixties and all the years beyond, they counsel, advise, share experiences, and act as mentor or resident wise ones to those who feel they need help.

Who will come to us for wise counsel?

1. Not fools. Fools already "know everything" or imagine they

do. Fools always imagine that they are wise and that the wise ones themselves are the fools.

Also, let's not forget that some older persons are also fools. They never did wise up.

2. Other older persons who are wise enough to know they need the special wisdom of a friend will come. Not all older persons are wise experts who can counsel others, but they are wise enough to recognize wisdom in another, and as necessary they will come for counsel.

3. Children will come for counsel. Grandchildren, teenagers, top young students who are planning ahead, children in conflict, children in fear and abuse, children in problem families—all of these will come to one who has the three reputations (a reputation for wisdom, a reputation for willingness to share, and a reputation for friendliness).

4. Teens, young adults, and adults in crisis will come.

5. Wise persons will come for counsel! The wiser one is, the more he will search out the wise counsel of others.

What questions are asked of a wise person? Answer: questions about life, all the questions wise persons have asked themselves.

1. Questions about romance: Does he love me? Does love come back after it has ebbed away? What is true love? How can I know if I love her?

2. Questions about parenting.

3. Questions about bad habits and inner conflicts.

4. Questions about purpose and meaning, human existence, God's nature, God's plan, and God's forgiveness.

5. Questions about friendship.

6. Questions about old age, dying, and death.

7. Questions about employment, money, and business.

How does a wise person answer?

1. He answers only after much listening. He is a great listener because he knows the danger of advising before all the relevant facts are before him.

2. She asks many questions before she answers. This is to acquaint herself with all the relevant facts.

3. He suppresses in himself all of his theories of personality and human nature. The wise person recognizes that humans are more different than they are the same, so book learning about psychology is only of limited value in counseling. "This person who has come to me for help is unique, so I must get his story—his history —and my counsel must be uniquely for him."

4. The wise woman answers with caution. "Fools rush in where angels fear to tread." The wise woman is never overconfident, never certain. The answers are never obvious, never easy, and never simple. "Life is so very complicated, so think about my advice for a few days before you act on it. Take time to decide if what I have said applies to your life. Remember, I only know a very small percentage of what there is to know about you. There is always the possibility that there is a better way than I have suggested, so think carefully before you take my advice."

5. The wise man often says, "I don't know the answer to that question; perhaps the two of us together can look for some answers for you."

6. The wise woman often says, "I can't help you with this because I do not know enough about it, but perhaps my friend or colleague Miss So-and-So can help you. May I call her and ask for you?"

There is another question to be answered briefly before leaving the subject of wisdom: What is the relation of wisdom to joy? We answered this question previously, but we repeat the answer briefly. Joy is the goal of so much we do, but it is an emotion that evades us if we pursue it directly. Rather than pursue joy directly, we must pursue the qualities of life that lead to joy. Wisdom is the first of the many qualities of character and personality that tend to lead to joy.

Wisdom is no guarantee of joy, but it greatly increases the probability of joy. One reason that age fifty-five to sixty-five is the happy time of life is that persons of this age are much wiser than before. They know much more, and they apply this knowledge in the management of their lives. Bill has for years been in the rough and tough of the construction business with all of its up-and-down cycles, moving about to find work, and a job where wisdom is critical. At age sixty-one Bill says, "At last I really have a handle on my life and my work; I really can manage my needs, my emotions, and my self-control. In my work pressures I can make a good decision. I can handle conflicts between the men; I can say no to an opportunity for a big profit because I know the opportunity, as good as it is, would overextend my resources and my men. No wonder I am a happy person: I have reduced the frustrations and the fears of my job. I actually enjoy the pace and the challenges because I am so much more realistic. I mean, I no longer exaggerate the opportunities; I no longer preoccupy myself with the negatives. I call it the way it is—*A* is *A*—and things work out in a pleasant atmosphere." Wisdom tends to lead to joy, as it did for Bill, but there is no guarantee.

A Good Heart

Good in this expression means "goodness and virtue," and *heart* means our "disposition and attitude" toward others. A good heart means that we treat others in a just and fair way, and our attitude is one of kindness and concern.

Higher life satisfaction goes hand in hand with a good heart. Those in the happy time of life are happy in part because they have a good heart. The good heart comes first, and the happiness follows. The good heart of middle age is more mellow. We do mellow with age, and the harsh and rigid ideals of youth soften. There is a more gentle attitude to the weaknesses and failings of others. Character weakness is understood by older persons who tend to criticize less often and to pass judgment less often. They tend to look for solutions instead of dwelling on the horror of the sin. Older persons remember their own weaknesses, and they usually see little benefit in casting the first stone. They look for a remedy, not a penalty. They want to turn a negative into a positive. They would rather say a kind, constructive word than say a hurtful one.

No wonder those who have a good heart are happier: they have fewer enemies! Their disposition makes friends, not enemies.

Their goodness tends to turn enemies into friends, and it tends to make good friends better friends. Who needs fighting and bickering over differences of opinion? Isn't there a middle road of compromise that can heal the breach? Let's sit at the bargaining table a little longer, and perhaps we will find a way for both sides to win. Let's bury the hatchet, but not in somebody's back.

On the other side of the coin, a good heart is happier because it does take a strong stand for fairness and kindness in certain situations. Then, when others' feathers are ruffled and they feel unkindly toward us, at least we can live with ourselves afterward because we remember we did take the right stand. Compromise is not the answer to everything, and a good heart knows it is necessary at times to declare what side you are on and then stand up and be counted. A major part of happiness is being able to live with your inner self in peace and self-respect, and a good heart is certainly a step toward inner peace and self-respect.

A good heart, then, tends to be a stepping-stone to happiness. Our goodness, fairness, justice—all of these earn the respect and affection of others. Their respect for us increases our self-respect, and there is in us a spiral of happiness that increases as goodness grows.

Meaningful Relationships

A meaningful relationship is understood and appreciated for what it is. Relationships increase in satisfaction as our understanding of relationships increases. We must understand the *basis of attraction* in relationships. We must also have skill in *identifying and resolving conflicts* in relationships. We must also accept the *limitations* of relationships. If we fail in any of these, then relationships tend to be frustrating. Success in dealing with attraction, conflicts, and limitations tends to encourage relationships to continue in a meaningful way. A major source of life satisfaction in "the happy time" is meaningful relationships.

Think for a moment about relationships among the young. The inexperience of the young can only be remedied by experience— good old trial-and-error experience—where it is often necessary to learn the hard way. Twenty-four-year-old Betty asks, "Do I love him, or is this friendship? What do I admire about him? What does he admire about me? Does he love me? If so, will his love ebb or flow? What can I do to make his love increase? What should I do with my anger toward him about his attitude (or finances or goals or habits or whatever)?" Betty asks the questions, but it may take her decades of living to find the answers. It will take her decades of living to manage relationships so they develop in a meaningful way.

Bernice, age fifty-seven, has been through these decades of experimental living; she has earned her diploma from the school of hard knocks, and consequently she has a good grasp of the different basis of relationships, the various alternatives of conflict resolution, and the limitations of relationships. These three relationship skills help her to manage her part of the marriage, her part in her friendships, her part in her business and social associations, and her part in her family relationships. Not that things are perfectly idyllic, but the relationships are meaningful and give her a great deal of life satisfaction. Not that she could discuss the relationships in terms of theory; she couldn't. But she survives in her relationships and derives the satisfaction that comes from meaning.

Noble Adventures—The Icing on the Cake

Noble adventures add challenge and excitement to the happy times. It is not enough to have calmness, inner peace, satisfaction, and meaning. The sparkle and the freshness of relevant living is important, too, and this often comes from hitching your life to a great project of spiritual, moral, religious, or humanitarian value. The joyful persons are often those who have found a project, cause, institution, crisis, human need, or opportunity, and they pour their resources, wisdom, and energy into the furtherance and enhancement of their project. These are the people who are living life today to its fullest, for whom life is a veritable celebration.

What are some examples of noble adventures that add challenge and excitement to living?

1. Charlie decided that the volunteer workers in the Legion were in need of help, and Charlie reorganized them and helped in the sick visitation, financial distributions, and general leadership of the branch. His energy over the years was phenomenal, and his very real contribution earned him an honorary life membership and the appreciation and respect of every branch member. But what it gave Charlie was new vigor, self-respect, challenge, and a new lease on life. Noble adventures normally provide this kind of stimulation. Good-bye boredom!

2. Let's recall Eula, the widow and sole supporter of four children. Remember her great project of her second half of life. Eula, age sixty-two, knew that one adventure was more noble than all the rest, and she wanted to participate in this noble adventure. Bold Mission Thrust was her denomination's home and foreign mission focus, and it led Eula to Africa, where she celebrated life hour by hour in the activities of a village mission station in Tanzania. The years went by, and she continued in a state of humble service in a noble adventure that captivated her heart and soul.

3. Orville, age fifty-nine, did it differently. He found a dingy hundred-year-old abandoned church building in a downtown slum, and on his own initiative he arranged purchase of the building, renovations and financing through a heritage fund, and structural repairs through a core initiative grant. A young seminarian graduated from Berkeley and came to pastor this downtown ministry, and Orville, the man from the right side of the tracks, was the seminarian's support in literally dozens of different ways.

4. What will your great project be for the second half of life? You may have more than one. Be prepared for the excitement coming your way. Religious activities, social activities that focus on critical needs of special groups, organized minor league sports, health care, educational projects, service to the handicapped, political contributions, employment projects—what will be your area of service?

5. Many employers, business managers, and executives manage

their business as though it were a sacred trust, a calling of God;
and this makes their business that noble adventure which is the
exciting reason for their existence. Many church members serve
in whatever positions fulfill them, and this is the heart and soul
of their existence in the second half of life. They ask themselves
rhetorically, "What could ever bring more joy of living than faithful service in a New Testament congregation?" Many persons
help a family member, a friend, or a neighbor in major significant
ways, and this helping relationship is their noble adventure.
What is your noble adventure?

6. There is another type of noble adventure where a person sees
the goal as being the best possible person. Living and doing one's
best becomes the noble adventure. Can you become excited about
being a good person? Many can, and they do the best they can,
brightening the small corner where they are. They brighten the
lives of their spouses, their children, their friends, their neighbors, and their congregations. Their life surely is a noble adventure.

Life-Style Has Its Own Rewards

Different life-styles bring different consequences for the years
from fifty-five to sixty-five. There are life-styles that prolong life
and multiply satisfactions, and there are life-styles that destroy.

How do the *physical factors* of life-styles affect our level of life
satisfaction? Proper diet, adequate exercise, rest, and a relaxed
approach to life all contribute to longevity and happiness. Many
of the overweight, sedentary, and Type A persons die from wrong
life-styles before they even reach the happy decade. Still others
have such a life-enhancing style that at age sixty they have the
mind and body of a person many years younger, and they are
ideally suited to live longer and enjoy life to its fullest.

How do the *mental, emotional, and social factors* affect our level
of life satisfaction? *Mental* factors include clear thinking, sound
reason, and sound values. *Emotional* factors include emotional
openness and honesty, a caring for others that must be combined
with a certain toughness or assertive attitude that leads us to

stand up for our rights without hurting others. *Social* factors that enhance the quality of life include friendliness, moderate expectations of others, and ability to enjoy our own company and pursue our own goals even while a part of a social group that pressures us to go its way. The happy decade is happy because most humans have sorted out their lives and made good choices about these factors. What are some of the special life-style factors that are of major importance for you to work on in the happy time? Let us list some of these factors:

(a) *Clear Thinking.* Clear thinking is a major source of higher life satisfaction. Much of the happiness of the happy decade can be traced back to good decisions that were arrived at by reason and logical thinking. Older persons know what they want (the goal), and they have learned *how to plan* those intermediate steps that will take them to their goal. Their plans are realistic, practical, and sensible; these plans have been formulated by the clear thinking of sound reason. No wonder these persons are happy—clear thinking has helped them to have the kind of life they want. But the irrational persons, whose feelings run their lives, never do find enduring life satisfaction.

(b) *Adequate Willpower.* Willpower is the ability to say no to short-lived pleasures for the sake of long-term advantages. Willpower opts for the long-term, not the short-term. Without willpower we flit here and there looking for momentary pleasures, and we never attain the enduring satisfactions. Willpower resists this temptation. Willpower makes tough, firm, and fair decisions, even if these decisions are unpopular.

(c) *Good Habits.* Those who are happiest in the happy decade are doing better at saying *no* to bad habits we have mentioned, including:

overweight	laziness	big spending
alcohol	moodiness	willfulness
nicotine	impulsiveness	shyness
drug abuse	procrastination	egotism
illicit sex	exhausting schedules	false pride
criminal activities	poor planning	violence

All of us have one or more bad habits that are robbing us of life satisfaction, and the important thing is to continue to get advice and to struggle against the bad habits with the best possible strategy. Identify your bad habits, and keep on struggling to break them.

(d) *Pacing Ourselves.* Our pace is also a habit. Listen as George says, "I enjoy the fact that the big rush is over. My pace is only half the speed it was ten years ago, but I'm getting more things accomplished. Hazel and I have time to enjoy ourselves; we have time to do things we enjoy." This saying "The hurrieder I go, the behinder I get" describes the hurrying of inexperience. The happiness of the second half of life is the opposite of hurrying and comes from first, slowing down,

then seeing things more clearly,

then making better decisions,

then getting more accomplished with much less effort.

Most of us do learn finally to slow down, and we learn that:

Perhaps a brisk walk is better than a run;

Perhaps a nap will refresh us and increase efficiency;

Perhaps if we don't do it, someone else will do it better;

Perhaps it needs to be left undone, so the need is more apparent.

Our own pace decreases; our efficiency and satisfaction increase.

At Peace with the Past

Every life has its share of heartaches and disappointments: loves lost, illness, death of family and friends, career setbacks, moral failures and indiscretions, injuries, misunderstandings, and persisting bad habits. The question is: "Will we cling to these hurts, or will we let them go?" Clinging to past hurts or letting them go—the choice is ours. It seems that the majority of those over fifty-five can let go, while a minority dwell on this host of negatives and then spoil their todays and tomorrows.

What are some helpful ways to let go of past heartaches and disappointments?

1. Force yourself to stop talking about past misfortunes and

mistakes. It is a mistake to talk about so many negatives because the talking revives and sharpens our memories and prevents the memory fading that is so helpful which comes from the passing of time. Let your past mistakes fade away. Talking about recent mistakes and new sins is helpful and important, so we can analyze the mistakes and learn our lesson. Talking about old mistakes and misfortunes is a scheme of self-pity that is intended to get us sympathy. This self-pity is not good for us as it means we are stranded or marooned in our past, and we are dead or unresponsive to present opportunities.

2. Learn to look at all of life—the good and the bad—as valuable learning. Life should be a school, and the beauty of learning a lesson from a mistake is that we can avoid making the same mistake again. Learn to use the lessons from past mistakes upon which to build a better life.

3. Stop thinking that your sufferings are unique, more intense, or more enduring. Join a group who have your same problems, handicaps, or weaknesses, and learn that there are many others worse off than you, and they are happily making the very best of their situation. "I felt so sorry for myself because I had no shoes, and then I met a boy who had no feet."

4. God is just as much involved in our failures as He is in our successes. He could easily have prevented each of our failures, but He knew we needed both—successes *and failures*—if we were ever going to mature. Learn the lesson of past mistakes, and then put past mistakes where they belong—behind you!

9

Growing Older— Age 65 and Up

The Dismal Facts of Old Age Are Opportunities

Our basic point throughout this book has been that the second half of life ought to be the better half. "Better" here means more meaningful and more joyful. "The better half" means that the middle years and old age and dying ought to be more meaningful and more joyful than the years of childhood and youth. As we have completed our analysis and study of the middle years, age forty-five to sixty-five, we should now appreciate the gradual and steady improvement that occurs in the quality of life throughout the middle years. Meaning and enduring joy do increase as the years pass because we have learned to live more effectively. Life is a good teacher, and we do learn how to live and achieve our goals and become the kind of person we want to be. This achievement and success brings joy.

The improvement of the middle years should not stop there. The learning about how to live should continue, and in old age we should become the real masters of the art of living. With mastery in the art of living should come the fullest joy. Joy is the fundamental universal emotion which signals that we are pleased with the way in which our life is progressing and unfolding. The ancient Roman senator Seneca was an avid supporter of the theory of the abundance of joy in old age when he remarked, "Life is most delightful when it is on the downward slope."

But to give this positive view of aging a basis in fact, and to avoid the fantasies and illusions of exaggeration and one-sidedness, we need to face the dismal facts of old age. Facts are facts, whether they are dismal or encouraging, and facts should be faced with intellectual honesty, so we can be certain that we are moving in the right direction. There are many encouraging facts of old age, which we will look at in detail. Let's be fair and honest and look at the dismal facts. What are the dismal facts of old age, and is there a way that dismal facts can be turned into opportunities?

Dismal Fact Number One

Ill health increases with age. This means that all of our bodily functions—our vision, hearing, breathing capacity, heart function, liver and kidney function, brain function—become less and less efficient with advancing age. We will be making more visits to the doctor's office.

Attitude is important about ill health. The best attitude is the one that says, "I will be health conscious to a reasonable degree, seeking to extend and maintain my health as much as possible. I will cooperate with medical advice and have regular checkups. I will accept the decline of health and vigor when I cannot change it, but I will *not* accept the decline if medical help and appropriate improvements in my life-style can reverse it."

Dismal Fact Number Two

Many friends and family will move away or die. Things will not stay the same; they will be different. If you make a list of the important people in your life, the names will change often. Meaningful relationships, though, can become more meaningful with age because we know more and more about meaning and friendship.

So this dismal fact challenges us to make one new friend a year—deliberately planning to have replacement friends for those who die or move away or fade away. This somewhat calculated strategy will keep a rich number of meaningful relationships in our life to the end. Can a calculating strategy bring joy?

Certainly it can, and a new friend a year is an example of strategy that leads to joy. Work at it.

When Peter died, Madge was on her own. Children and grandchildren were too far away to see often. She joined the Seniors club and was soon participating in many activities with people her own age, in the same financial circumstances and with the same physical capabilities. Arranged theater trips, shopping trips, indoor sports, and musical programs opened new doors of enjoyment. She made new friends who had gone through a similar loss of spouse and lifetime companion and could identify with her loneliness and aloneness.

Dismal Fact Number Three

Old roles exit, and we are always just a year away from no roles at all. Roles are tasks, jobs, responsibilities, positions. We enjoy roles because they give us status, honor, and regular activities that relate us closely to those around us. But roles change too, especially at retirement, or when we move or when we have health problems. As roles exit, we should have a roving eye for new roles that we can seek out and obtain for ourselves. Find a new role a year to add to our new friend a year!

This short list of dismal facts covers the main negatives of old age. The facts are dismal, but each one is an opportunity in disguise. It is what we do with each dismal fact that has a negative or a positive bearing on our life. If we respond to a dismal fact positively, making the best of the situation, then the dismal fact is not for us. The dismal facts of old age are not for the person who turns them into an opportunity. Are you a person who lets things get you down, or do you struggle and overcome? Strategy is the key, and careful planning and long-term strategy are vital to take the "dismal" out of the facts of old age.

The Exciting, Encouraging, Unlimited Possibilities Ahead!

Look back a little—to see where you have come from and to evaluate what you did. But then look ahead a lot. You have just crossed the great divide from middle age into old age, and the possibilities ahead are exciting, encouraging, and unlimited. Look ahead, because you have herewith a lot of planning to do.

Age sixty-five is usually our great divide, although not always so. Certainly old age begins at a different time for every person. Some retire at fifty-five, and these have made the adjustment to a new life by age sixty, while others retire at other ages, and still others never do retire. The age of retirement, whether sixty-five or another year, is a year of unequaled opportunity. The opportunity is the choices we can make concerning all the options and alternatives that present themselves for all our remaining years. Think of the size of this opportunity in terms of the probable length of your old age. Assuming you retire when many do at age sixty-five, and if you live to eighty, this gives you fifteen years of old age. That is a big block of time available for you in the prime of your life.

Retire at	Estimated Length of Life	Available years
Age 65	Age 80	15 years
Age 65	Age 85	20 years
Age 65	Age 90	25 years
Age 65	Age 95	30 years
Age 60	Age 95	35 years

What are you going to do with the next twenty-five years of your life? Plan, make a new start, and get ready to do a lot more living.

Good planning for old age must begin with an assessment of the possibilities. How great are the possibilities? They are as wide as our imagination and our courage. These two qualities—imagination and courage—help us to assess the possibilities and see the full range of the opportunities ahead. Imagination is capable of letting our minds wander over the full range of our interests, capabilities, and resources. Imagination also opens our vision to the possibilities for involvement in our own village, our own city street and apartment block, or involvement in activities across town or in another state, province, country, or continent. For many of us the world is our limit, and that is what is so exciting about old age. But often the greatest opportunity is next door or just down the road.

After imagination comes courage, which challenges us to do new things, not just the same old safe things we have done before. Courage involves facing danger and risk. Courage means we control our fears, and we venture toward the unknown, not recklessly but with the wisdom of a lifetime guiding us. There are not many noble adventures of old age that would ever begin without a large amount of courage. Excitement and challenge is unknown in old age if we do not make courageous decisions.

Jack and Alice had never ventured further than the cottage or the lake in forty years of marriage. Now they had decided to go on a safari in Africa. Friends and relatives thought they were crazy, but they had screwed up their courage and "taken up the challenge."

After this first trip, which opened up a whole new life, Jack and Alice spent many happy hours planning their next trip. Before Jack's death they were able to take four wonderful tours, which they wouldn't have done if they hadn't put aside their fears and found the courage to take the first trip.

Another aspect of looking ahead comes when we view old age as a new beginning. Because we age slowly and it takes a long time to arrive, we may forget that old age is something new for us. Because it is new, it deserves a proper beginning. Let's make old age a new beginning. Let's approach it as a new adventure, largely unaffected by past commitments, mistakes, or interests. Old age deserves a brand-new start, with the hopefulness that is only fair to grant to a new adventure.

As we look ahead, what shall we do about Hollywood's gloomy view of old age? Can Hollywood, the youth culture, and commercialism be wrong about the second half of life? Can it be that their negative view of old age as a hopeless, joyless, senseless decay and withering has missed the whole point? Of course they are wrong and have missed the point, and the reasons are heartbreaking. First, some older persons are wasting and withering in a pathetic old age that is void of imagination and courage, and their empty lives have triggered the gloomy view of aging.

Second, commercialism aims its flattery, deception, false values, and social pressures at young people more than older persons because the young tend to part with their money more easily, and the older persons hang on to theirs. The older persons know a smooth-talking con job when they see one, whether it is a medicine man with a horse and wagon or a drug company selling painkillers on prime time TV. The older persons have been stung before. Once stung, twice shy. Older persons recognize flattery and deception, while younger persons buy the products they don't need or can't afford. No wonder the media pipes a tune to lure the young. It is not the joy of youth, but rather the incompleteness of youth that leads youth to fall for commercialism. "Perhaps this new shirt or coat or car will make me more of a man," says the young person, and the car manufacturer or coat maker says, "Yes, it certainly will."

The possibilities of old age truly are exciting, encouraging, and unlimited. With good planning, imagination, courage, and a refusal to accept the false views of the youth cult, older persons can find meaning and joy in abundance in the years of their seventies, eighties, nineties, and beyond.

It is just recently that older people have been used on TV commercials. Now old-time movie stars supplement their fading bank accounts by touting everything from dog food to hemorrhoid relievers. Consumers can relate to a person in his sixties advertising a product for arthritis more so than someone of twenty pushing the same products. Manufacturers, advertisers, and public relations people have realized the number and the buying power of seniors and are catering to them more.

The fountain of youth is now challenged by the wave of gray!

What Are You Going to Do for the Next Twenty-five Years?

That is right: twenty-five years more. You say, "I'll never make it, and I don't even know if I want all that time." The fact is that you may very well have twenty-five years or more, but whatever time you have left, twenty-five years or twenty-five weeks, good planning can multiply the exciting possibilities ahead.

1. We have discussed *"a new friend a year."* But new friends have to be found. Go looking for them. Get out where there are people. Set *two days a week aside* for meeting new people and doing things with groups of people. That is one hundred days a year for getting out of the house. It is every fourth day seeing new faces in a planned effort to make a new friend a year. Remember: You probably have still not met your very best friend, so go looking for him or her or them.

2. We have also discussed *"a new role a year."* Get out some newspapers and cut clippings of many activities which older persons are enjoying. Make a list of possible roles for you. The list should be very long because the world is full of stories of older persons enjoying very unique and meaningful roles. In fact, this generation of older people is accepting a much wider range of exciting responsibilities and activities. You don't need to live in "dull city"—as the new expression says it. At whatever your age, there are things to do that can enrich every day beyond your highest hopes. No matter how many exciting roles you find and accept, save some energy and time for Bold Mission Thrust.

3. Another planning possibility is *"four or more major moves in old age."* Many older persons and older couples find it very acceptable to make *one* retirement move, and they make this major move with the right attitude of hopeful anticipation. But when the move is not a permanent solution, and they do not find all they want that move to be, they remain mentally "frozen" in that dream instead of letting imagination and courage lead them to get moving to a better arrangement. The better arrangement may be just a modification of the original dream, but they should pursue that modificiation.

Some do find that one retirement move is enough, but many others need to make more moves—to move to Florida, then move back home, and then move back to Florida again for four months a year, and finally move to a seniors' villa back home. That is four moves!

It is not practical to expect that one move can be enough for all of us, and some may move quite a few times in their search for the best accommodation and environment. Listen to Gus and Marge: "Well, we lived back East away from our children and grandchildren. We dreamed for years of moving West to be closer to the kids. But when we did move there, we missed our old friends; we disliked the weather, and we got a bigger dose of our children and grandchildren than we needed. So move number two saw us back East for the summers only to avoid the heat of the west. Move number three saw us back in the West year round in an air-conditioned seniors' villa with friends from the East coming to visit, and us making occasional trips to see them."

Listen to Ruth: "I was desperate when Harold died because I was afraid to live alone. First, I sold the house and moved to an apartment five minutes' drive from my youngest son. This was a good move for me at the time, and I stayed there three years. By then, at age seventy-one and in good health, I knew I would enjoy a senior citizens' complex, so after much searching, I found what I thought would be a pleasant place. It turned out to be a perfect spot. I made my own meals, got out often, and made good friends.

"Eight years later, when I was seventy-nine, both of my daughters asked me to consider moving closer to them, so I moved out of province to a retirement place where I have my own small suite. I eat my meals in a beautiful cafeteria, but I can cook in my suite if I choose to do so. This has lasted three years. I am delighted to be age eighty-two, and I'm delighted my family sees me every day or else phones. One of my daughters is pressing me to move in with them, and I may just do it if I can persuade her and her husband to let me keep some of my independence, privacy, and my own activities. They know I like to be busy, and that I will get out and join the organizations I prefer, and they seem to think they would enjoy having me."

Ruth is another example of a person who made a number of major moves in old age, always seeking improvements but making moves wisely.

Begin with Life-Changing Decisions

Not to make a decision is a decision too. It's a decision by default, but it is still a decision. "I am planning a great old age," said Hector, but nothing ever came out of Hector's planning because he never made any decisions. An exciting old age can only come about as we make life-changing decisions, such as:

1. To retire or not to retire. One third of all males over age sixty-five are employed. What is your choice? Many find that the decision to retire is the decision to die, and one or two or three years later they do die of physical malfunctions that can be traced to inactivity, overeating, and stress. Do you have a choice of retirement? If you don't have a choice, and the decision is made for you, then focus on what to do in your retirement. Retirement is the opportunity par excellence which opens the door to a whole new world. If you have the choice of retiring, then consider it seriously, and consider if you could reduce your work week instead of continuing full-time. Many of us, because we want to work, should work throughout our lives with a lessening work load with advancing age.

2. How shall I invest my wisdom, resources, and energy in the service of my ideals? What do I believe in, and *who* do I believe? What should be my commitment to my values—my religious faith? How can I implement this? How can older persons best promote their own visions of a better world?

3. How shall I relate to my family in the years to come? Shall we move across the country to be closer to our sons/daughters/grandchildren?

4. What new projects and adventures shall I begin?

5. What habits do I need to break?

6. How shall I make new friends?

7. What new roles shall I accept?

8. What habits do I need to start?

9. What obstacles in my mind (wrong values, wrong beliefs, or wrong attitudes) stand in the way of a much better old age?

Once again imagination and courage are needed to make the

decisions that need to be made, and to imagination and courage should be added the trademark of old age: wisdom.

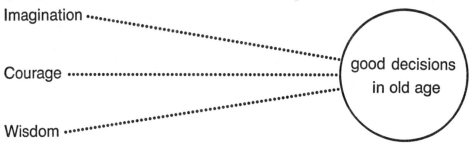

Share Your Wisdom, or Miss the Point

This important point is repeated: either your old age includes opportunities to share your wisdom with others, or you have missed the central function and purpose of old age. The first half of life is more for self: finding self and getting self going well. The second half of life is more for others:

sharing one's wisdom with others,

sharing one's love and affection with others,

sharing one's resources with others,

sharing the truths of life as we have come to know them.

This sharing includes development of *the three reputations:*

1. A reputation for being wise.
2. A reputation for willingness to share our wisdom.
3. A reputation for friendliness.

As we cultivate these reputations for ourselves, people will want to come to ask us our advice.

In addition to the three reputations, we also need to be willing to accept help and friendship from those who are younger. Shame on those old persons who, in their fierce desire to be independent and not be a burden, turn down offers of help from the young. This is bad strategy, and the younger persons take our desire for independence and privacy as a wish not to be involved. The wiser way is to accept the offers of help mainly as a way to let relationships develop. Out of these relationships we earn the confidence and trust of the young, and then they come to us for counsel, encouragement, and friendship. The most beautiful words from the elderly are not "No thank you, I can manage all right," but rather, "Yes, thank you so much for the offer of your help. Let me do my share too, but it will be so much nicer with the two of us doing it together. I love the help, and I love the company. And how are things going with you?" Let yourself be involved in the lives of younger people in the only way they know to approach you, namely, by offering you some help on your way. Then the relationship has a mutual attraction.

Wisdom is the strength of old age, and physical strength is the power of youth. What better way to bind the generations together than to let each generation benefit from the other generations! This is the way it ought to be. Also, what is the matter with *asking for help?* Older persons can take the initiative and ask for help, and this becomes a signal and example to others that they too can ask older persons for help. "Older persons without younger persons blow away; younger persons without older persons blow up." So get together, generations!

Use It or Lose It:
Arguments for a Very Active Life-Style

This point was made much earlier but for emphasis must be repeated: Joyful living comes from being physically, mentally, emotionally, and socially active. Happiness in old age comes from struggling to keep active as long as possible. Activity is an elixir that leads to happiness. Don't worry about wearing out from activity because rusting out through inactivity is the much greater danger. Don't sit staring at TV or out the window. Fill your life with meaningful activity.

Be active all your life in your congregation and other organizations. Make friends, accept new roles, and find social responsibilities.

Be active physically—working or exercising. Sit, stand, walk, do your gardening, housekeeping, house repairs, yard work, car repairs—as long as you can. Shape up the old body, and keep it in shape by moderate exercise.

Your brain desperately needs work too! Keep your brain in top form by giving it work to do. Just fifteen minutes per day of memory exercises will keep your memory in good form. Read, study, think, debate, learn, solve problems, and your brain will serve you well as long as you live. Old brains are better—if they have exercise. Constant exercise of mental faculties is essential to keep the brain at its best.

Roll with the Punches, or Get Hurt

There is a strategy in the sport of boxing called rolling with the punches, meaning that you can lessen the blow of the punch by moving backward slightly as the blow hits. If you roll backward, and there is some rhythm to your movement, you can swing in the same direction as the punch as soon as you see it coming. Do you roll with the punches of life, that hit the heart, the pocketbook, the soul, the self-confidence, and the stamina? Or does your rigidity or false pride or lack of readiness or preoccupation with other things mean you have to "take it straight on the chin"? Many good boxers have made the mistake of taking it on the chin and, as a consequence, they have gone down and lost the fight.

In youth and middle age there is still lots of time left to recover from losses, so losses are less serious. To lose one's lifesavings at age thirty-five is not the same as losing one's savings at age seventy-five. Rolling with the punches means you don't set yourself up so any one single punch can flatten you. To avoid one fatal punch to your pocketbook, spread your money around in a half-dozen good investments. Don't have all your "eggs" in one basket. To avoid one fatal punch to your social life, make sure you have more than one or two good friends. Only one or two meaningful roles is another danger; it is wiser and safer to work to maintain at least a half-dozen roles.

Another aspect of rolling with the punches is that you responded to the punch: you "rolled" with it, and your response means you admit you did get hit and that you are hurting. Emotional honesty means we admit we are hurting; we open up and share the experience. We don't deny it happened. In fact, if the hit has hurt us badly we holler ouch! by sharing the experience of pain with significant others. Debbie, age 78, was hurting deeply as the moving van pulled up to the farmhouse where she had lived fifty-two years. She watched for a while, with tears, as the movers loaded her life's possessions. Then she drove over to the neighbors and got some good-bye hugs and kisses. Debbie let the tears flow and honestly admitted her regrets about leaving the farm. The tears and the honesty about her regrets were her way of rolling with the punches, and in the evening as she sniffed the newness of her apartment and as she enjoyed the view from her window, she knew the decision was right. Her pain would be replaced by contentment and satisfaction.

Enjoy the Other Elderly

Every generation has an instinctive preference for itself, and the elderly are no exception. Older persons very much need their peers, and they need identification with the other elderly. Perhaps it is the similarity of past experience: "You know we all were in high school when the Great Depression hit." Perhaps it is the similarity of opportunity: "Sure, I can go golfing with you fellows three mornings a week." Perhaps it is the similarity of interests: "Yes, I am past the tennis stage, but I really enjoy a long walk." Whatever the reasons, older persons enjoy the conversation, comradeship, and companionship of other elderly. An important aspect of finding old age to be an enjoyable experience is the active pursuit of friendship and love with others who are old.

Encourage your congregation to have age-related activities for study, fellowship, and commitment. What a means of congregational outreach to have special ministries to the elderly.

Death of a Spouse

Is there life after death—after the death of a spouse, that is? Marriage is the deepest, most complicated, and most satisfying of all human relationships, and the death of a spouse is the greatest human emotional pain and distress. In old age, death of a spouse is even more distressing. In the middle of this loss of spouse, when we are blindly and numbly making our way through the gloom of funeral arrangements, and as we are in shock and disbelief in the weeks that follow, with lawyers to visit, estates to be settled, and many letters to write, we think only occasionally of the years and/or decades ahead. But three months later, on average, the curtain begins to lift, and we find ourselves looking ahead more and looking back less. The mind pursues its own healing, and the scars of the loss of our other half have formed, and suddenly we can look ahead. What a beautiful thing, this inner healing, this three-month period of recovery! On the day of the death of our spouse, all was hopeless; and three months later we can sense the beginning of a new energy and an inner rebuilding and recovery.

Yes, there is definitely life ahead after death of a spouse. But there is more difficulty ahead, more barriers to be removed than single persons experience in old age. The advantage of being single is that single persons have already adjusted to living alone before their old age; they know the importance of working harder at keeping an active roster of friends; and they have deliberately developed satisfying hobbies and projects which are important to them. The widow or widower is usually quite a few steps behind because married life tended to be fulfilling, and this meant other interests were left undeveloped. After the death of a spouse, it is important that the survivor make a major effort to build friendships, hobbies, and projects. This amounts to restructuring most of one's life, and this encompassing change is not without some stress and some reluctance to let go of the habits and patterns which were shaped by many years of marriage. But the marriage is over, and pleasant marital memories are *not* enough upon which to build a future. Do not let the memories of a beautiful marriage rob you of ten, twenty, or thirty years of joyful living in old age. Memories are not enough. It is life today and tomorrow that counts.

God Is So Good

God is involved—totally involved—in every human life, and His involvement is always wise, loving, and just. He is a helping, concerned, and faithful friend to every one of His adopted children, which we are if we accept His purpose and plan for us. God is never unjust, never uncaring, and never unkind. The full extent of God's love is revealed in Jesus Christ.

No one can know and appreciate the truth of God's goodness as well as an older person who has walked for many years the walk of faith. Older persons have the advantage of a longer time to experience the goodness of God. Older persons ought to know Him better because they have walked with Him longer.

At fifty and sixty years of age we should know beyond a doubt that God is good, based on our personal experience of our life. But when we reach seventy and eighty, and we are more certain than ever that God is, then, another element moves into focus—the fact of our death and our final liberation into God's eternal presence. How can we help but sense a growing anticipation of the enjoyment of His presence and an excitement about all that God has promised and planned for us when we join Him on the other side. With advancing age we enjoy the fact that fewer and fewer years and hours separate us from our great day with God.

10

Growing Old with a Positive Outlook

Attitude Is Everything

"Attitude is everything," says a popular song, and if this is an overstatement, then certainly attitude is at least a major significance. By attitude we mean a person's general frame of mind and hopes for the future. Attitudes can be positive or negative. What is your attitude? What is the best attitude for old age? Compare your attitude with these true statements about attitude:

1. "My happiness depends mainly on myself, not on government, not on agencies, not on the weather, not on chance, and not on circumstances. I need to think clearly, make good decisions, struggle to do my best, stand up for myself, be considerate of others, and pursue wisely what I want. Then my life will have the greatest likelihood of leading to happiness and joy."

2. "When others are negative, and when disappointments and setbacks occur, I have no choice but to reassess my situation and to get moving ahead again with energy and wisdom."

3. "I know how good life can be, and I know how unpleasant life can be. Whatever the circumstances, my responsibility is to pursue my ideals and my hopes with energy, wisdom, and patience as long as I can."

Growing Old with Self-Esteem

Do you know that we create our own character? Character is not something we are born with, and character is not given to us by childhood experience. Character comes from a thousand choices we make over the many years of childhood and adulthood as we are deciding on the kind of person we would like to be. In fact, each of us has the character—beliefs, values, attitudes, and personal style—that we have chosen for ourselves out of all the possible characters and character traits we have observed in our lifetime. It is an exciting and awesome thought that we are the kind of person we are because that is the kind of person we have chosen and choose to be. Character is not a passive happening; it is the sum and conclusion of a thousand choices about values, beliefs, attitudes, and lifestyle.

Not only do we create our own character, but we continually change, reshape, and strengthen our character throughout our life span. Character is not fixed and frozen forever in its only form. Examples of character change are any personal growth and upward revision of personal values, changes in beliefs, breaking of bad habits, learning of good habits, and changes of attitude. Not only can character change, but our whole lifetime is a conscious process of trying to improve and strengthen our character. Children, young adults, middle-aged adults, older adults—all of these are working on their character in a continuing process of trying to become a better person. Of course, as the years pass into old age, it is hoped that the task of character development is closer to being completed, and in most cases older adults are only "touching up" their character or working on the finishing touches of growth in character.

Self-esteem is the process of being pleased with the character we have created for ourselves. Self-esteem is liking your character. You take a look at yourself and the character you have created, and you decide you did a fairly good job on it. You are still working to improve your character—that is a lifelong task, but you can live quite well with it as is. Self-esteem means that we are pleased that our character strengths outweigh our character weaknesses. We tolerate the weaknesses while at the same time striving to turn them into character strengths.

Self-esteem has to be earned by keeping our character in good shape. Life on planet earth is a continuous contamination of character, and if we are not careful, our character goes backward: the mere process of living can see our beliefs, values, habits, and attitudes sliding downhill into an ugly selfishness, unkindness, ignorance, error, and prejudice. We have to be on our guard, or we will fall into bad habits and very unacceptable attitudes.

In old age, as we have slowly brought our character up to the highest level, it is all the more easy for us to slide backward. Older persons know very well how easy it is to be less than our best, and eternal vigilance of character and life-style is the cost of being the best person we can be. The physical weakness of old age means there is more struggle to just keep going through each day. This means there is less available energy to struggle to keep our behavior in line with our ideals. What a challenge it is to do what we know we ought to do when painful joints, weak legs, shortness of breath, unsteadiness on our feet, and a weakening sense of balance seem to be holding us back from doing our best. Growing old with self-esteem is costly, but most older adults are eager to pay the price and keep their self-esteem by the endless challenge of character maintenance and character growth.

Turning Four Negatives into Positives

The human mind is powerful, practical, and creative. When it cannot get us to make changes by means of rewards and pleasant outcomes, the human mind has a number of negatives by which it can pressure us to change. Four of these mental negatives are:
1. Depression
2. Anxiety
3. Loneliness
4. Boredom

The mind uses these four negatives to pressure us to make

necessary constructive changes in our life, especially changes in our thinking, attitudes, and life-style.

The	should lead	make	resulting	more
Four	⟶	personal change	⟶	joy in
Negatives	us to	of thinking	in	living
		and life-style		

The four negatives employ painful discomfort in the form of misery, frustration, restlessness, and anguish to motivate us to improve our life circumstances. Because of the usual positive outcomes of the four negatives, we say these negatives are actually positives in disguise. These negatives can lead to joy as we:

(a) Realize that depression, anxiety, loneliness, and boredom are reliable indicators of the need for personal changes.

(b) Realize that the four negatives are not the obstacles; the four negatives are the four great motivators to get us to remove the obstacles that are blocking the pathway to joy.

(c) The obstacles that have to be removed are usually: (1) negative attitudes, (2) lack of self-confidence, (3) shyness, (4) cautiousness, (5) introversion, and (6) bad habits. These *six obstacles* have to be removed if we are to progress toward joyful living.

(d) We need to work constructively with the four negatives, and they will help us to remove the six obstacles.

Most older persons learned much earlier in their lives how to use the four negatives to overcome obstacles. Those who still haven't learned how have some exciting life-changing discoveries to make. The four negatives—depression, anxiety, loneliness, and boredom—are not the problem; in fact, they are part of the solution. As we study the meaning of the four negatives in our own lives, we see the changes we must make, and we are motivated to make these changes.

The Bright Side of Depression

Depression is an unpleasant and sometimes horrible experience, bringing misery, frustration, restlessness, and anguish. But depression should lead to great personal benefits and advantages, or else we have missed its purpose. The purpose of depression is to focus our attention on the need for important changes to be made which are overdue. It is to the benefit and advantage of depressed persons to cooperate with their depression by accepting responsibility to reassess their character and life situations with a view to making changes. We overcome depression by accepting the need to make changes and then going ahead and making the changes. If you are depressed, have you pinpointed the specific changes you need to make in your character or in your life situation?

Depression is a natural prod to engage in serious self-analysis and personal problem solving. Henry was sixty-seven years old, and over several months of summer he had slowly and surely slipped into a depression in which he felt worthless and had no desire to go on living. His wife June said, "Henry, can I help? Am I the cause? What would you like?" As he didn't answer, she finished dressing, picked up her briefcase, and drove to her executive job. "How can this be happening to me?" Henry asked himself. "Why am I so down in spirits? For years I couldn't wait for retirement at age sixty-five. Now I can sit at home just as I planned to do, and I can read or go golfing or sleep in late. What is the matter with me that I no longer enjoy any of the things which I looked forward to for so long?" As the weeks went by, Henry sat in his chair staring into the yard, and he was able to take this complicated puzzle, put the pieces together, and make the changes to improve his mood and his life situation.

First, June and Henry had made great plans for their retirement, but neither of them had thought carefully about what Henry would do at home by himself for the six years before June's retirement. Whenever Henry looked ahead to that six years, he had mistakenly thought, "After forty-five years of steady employment, I will love the rest when retirement comes." But six months of retirement without June at home was all he enjoyed. Second, June loved her work and told Henry all about it every evening. It made Henry sick to hear about it because he was so envious of

June's busy and enjoyable day. Third, Henry felt himself aging steadily and was fearful of waiting four more years until June's retirement; he wanted things different *now* or at least soon. As quickly as Henry started to piece together what was troubling him, his mood started to lift. His mood lifted further as he and June talked it over and made interesting "interim" retirement plans for Henry. Henry's depression resolved itself completely as soon as he tentatively tried out these interim plans and found them to his liking.

Henry's resolution of his depression follows a common pattern:

1. The depression comes.

2. We look for a discrepancy between our expectations and our own life situation as a possible cause of the depression. We had expected such and such, but where is it? Why have our expectations been unfulfilled?

3. We see which it is that we need to change, either our expectations or our life situation or both.

4. We make whatever changes are necessary, and the depression lifts.

Eleanor's husband died; she grieved deeply but slowly recovered and began to look forward to her future. She had decisions to make and made them. However, she could not live with the decisions but would not say so. She became depressed. Only when her depression pressured her to serious self-analysis and consideration of her life situation did Eleanor begin to understand what further changes she needed to make. As she made these new decisions, her depression lifted.

Irene became depressed when she went to live with her son and daughter-in-law. She had had expectations about how it would be, but life in the new setting was not as she had anticipated. But instead of complaining or renegotiating, Irene kept herself smiling at others, appearing agreeable. She soon became depressed. Why depressed?—because she was so full of unexpressed frustration. Her depression only lifted when she talked over the situation, which resulted in real changes that were an improvement for everyone concerned.

Other types of depressions are resolved when we break bad habits. Still other depressions are resolved as we build up our self-confidence and try new activities, or as we make demands on others that result in more equitable relationships.

The second half of life will have its depressions, but each of these depressions is an opportunity in disguise which we must seize by making changes in our character and/or our life situation. The following situations can bring depression with them *if we do not respond wisely:*

A. Loss of family and friends by death.

B. Loss of self-esteem due to diminished bodily functions, for example, urinary incontinence, faltering memory, poor hearing, or paralysis.

C. Altered social roles.

D. Less income

E. Lack of an adequate life view.

F. Inhibitory personality.

Turning Anxiety into Motivation

The second negative that leads to joy is anxiety. The discomforts of anxiety include tension, nausea, dry mouth, sweaty palms, rapid pulse, uneasiness, panic, dizziness, weakness, and butterflies. What is the purpose of these unsettling physical signs? The purpose is to motivate us to take constructive action to safeguard and enhance a threatened aspect of our lives. Anxiety, in other words, is an adaptive useful life-serving response because of its motivational value. Anxiety does not always bring improvements, but anxiety ought to lead to constructive action, which in turn ought to lead to joy.

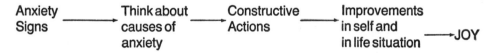

The discomforts of anxiety disappear when constructive action leads to improvement in self and life situations. This is a five-step process.

1. First come the discomforts of anxiety.

2. Then comes thinking, reasoning, and decisions about the possible source of the anxiety.

3. Now come constructive actions to change self and/or life situations.

4. This results in improvements in self and in life situations.

5. Finally comes a more contented, peaceful, and joyful state of mind.

Anxiety aims to reinforce and support our ideals and life goals. Anxiety is an effective motivator which arises when there is a conflict between our actual behavior and our life goals. These life goals are the goals and standards we have set for ourselves by which we can judge the quality of our own lives. As we are failing in our efforts to live by these goals and ideals, anxiety occurs and brings us back in the direction of our ideals. Anxiety commonly reminds us of the following life goals:

1. Survival, safety, comfort, and good physical health.

2. Proper diet, proper exercise, and proper rest.

3. Balanced attitude toward oneself (self-love, self-trust, and self-acceptance).

4. Realistic goals.

5. A satisfactory intimate relationship.

6. Good friendships.

7. Acceptable employment.

8. Emotional openness and honesty.

9. Fairness and kindness towards others.

10. Sense of meaning and purpose.

What if some of these goals are being jeopardized? Are we in some sort of danger because of our mistakes or unwise strategies and actions? Anxiety will result if our life goals are threatened. What is the only effective anxiety reducer? The only effective anxiety reducer is thinking, decisions, and a wise course of action that will safeguard and strengthen those life goals that are in danger.

Avoid the anxiety reducers that make the problem worse than before: alcohol, drugs, overeating, smoking, fighting, daydreaming, getting a headache, or cutting your wrist. All of these actions do produce temporary relief of anxiety which, however, is followed by bigger problems and worse anxiety.

Use moderately the anxiety reducers that provide temporary help: tapping your foot, concentrating on your navel or the tip of the nose, talking, physical exercise, deep breathing, talking about emotions, and sex.

Place your main emphasis on turning anxiety into motivation. The motivation should result in thinking, decisions, and actions that will strengthen and improve your life in those areas about which you are concerned.

Anxiety in old age tends to subside and is not as serious a problem. The peaks of anxiety are not as high as they were in youth, but the time required to return to lower anxiety is longer. The causes of anxiety in old age are the same as the causes in youth, namely, our indecision and/or wrong decisions about self and/or life situation. Behind the indecision and/or wrong decisions are usually the six obstacles mentioned earlier: (1) negative attitudes, (2) lack of self-confidence, (3) shyness, (4) cautiousness, (5) introversion, and (6) bad habits.

To track down the cause of your anxiety, be on guard to see if the six obstacles are the villains. The way over anxiety is to remove the obstacles, as difficult as this may be. Anxiety is a necessary, useful pressure that your own mind places on itself to remove the sources of anxiety.

Loneliness Means I Must Make Social Changes

Loneliness is an important adaptive pressure for us to change our life-styles. If it weren't for loneliness, we would all live like grizzly bears, content to sit by ourselves each in our own corner of the forest. Loneliness is not a problem in itself. Rather, loneliness is part of the solution, as it motivates us to make changes in our schedule so that more people are included in our lives.

Keith, age seventy-four, was very lonely, so he took up the

winter sport of curling and the summer sport of lawn bowling. Hazel, age eighty, was lonely, and her loneliness pushed her to move across town to be close to her daughter, which resulted in ten more years of real enjoyment for her.

Loneliness changes its meaning in old age from a longing for interaction and emotional attachment (which is the meaning of loneliness in youth) to a longing for interesting activities. We do the elderly a favor when we emphasize a variety of interesting activities and when we deemphasize constant involved interactions with others. Noninterpersonal activities are very enjoyable for the elderly. By "noninterpersonal" is meant any social activities which actively involve other people *casually,* including:

1. Going with a group for a bus ride.
2. Attending church, study groups, work projects, or sharing times.
3. Going fishing with casual acquaintances.
4. Having coffee with a neighbor.
5. Spouse activities of routine nature, that is, shopping, household chores, and doctor's appointment.
6. Attending hobby classes and groups such as ceramics, music, photography, and gardening.
7. Attending any educational activities.
8. Helping a neighbor with car repairs, gardening, or house maintenance.
9. Cooking for a bake sale.
10. Employment in any amount.
11. Volunteer work.

Noninterpersonal activities should be:

A. Stimulating: physically, mentally, and socially.

B. Regular: Too much time between activities may mean our social skills get rusty.

C. Enjoyable: interesting, entertaining, intriguing, novel, and exciting.

"Loneliness means I must make social changes." Loneliness is usually caused by the six obstacles: negative attitude, shyness, lack of self-confidence, cautiousness, introversion, and bad habits.

Do something about overcoming these obstacles, and you will be on your way to enjoyable involvement and leaving loneliness behind. Let your loneliness motivate you to change, enrich, and expand your social life.

Boredom Means Many Things

Boredom is a serious problem for those elderly persons who are not really pursuing what they want. They don't have satisfying experiences because they do not pursue them. They have stopped struggling, or stopped investigating, or stopped living exuberantly, and the well of interesting, challenging adventures has dried up.

The underlying cause of boredom is often one of the following:

A. *Emotional inhibition and depression.* Many people are bored because they are depressed. They try to get interested in something, but their depression gets in the way. Unexpressed anger is often the basis of depressions that result in boredom. The only answer for this type of boredom is to resolve the depression by means of working through the anger.

B. *Wanting the impossible.* Some people are bored because they are wanting what is unattainable. Their finances or health will not allow their dreams to come true, so they live in frustration, pouting, and boredom. They need to revise their expectations downward to reality.

C. *Cautiousness.* A number of persons are bored because they have not enlarged their sphere of activity and opportunity due to cautiousness. In fact, their routine and environment are almost void of stimulation because over the years they have made wrong decisions and declined to expand their horizons. They must overcome boredom by daring to take the risk involved in new adventures, new hobbies, and new projects.

D. *Introversion.* "Nothing interests me except my own thoughts, reading, television, and one or two friends." We need to enrich our inner selves but not at the expense of an interesting and challenging social life. In general, most elderly persons should struggle to maintain a rich social experience.

E. *Blackmail*. Some boredom is not boredom at all: it is black-mail. This comes when a person tries to obtain favors and advantages unfairly by pressures such as guilt tripping or threats. "There is nothing to do in this place" may simply be a pressure ploy for more favors. We do blackmailers a service by never playing into their hands. Boredom should always be analyzed carefully as a problem to be solved. The answers are as varied as life itself.

11

The Closing Years— Depending on Others

Giving Up Independence

The first four stages of the second half of life involve living independently, and we have considered and described these four independence stages as:

1. Mid-Life Crisis—Ages 35 to 45
2. The Productive Years—Ages 45 to 55
3. The Happy Time—Ages 55 to 65
4. Growing Older—Age 65 and Up.

We have looked at each of these four stages to see what beliefs, attitudes, and goals can make each stage a better time through which to live.

The fifth and sixth stages of the second half of life require the help of others, and these stages are:

5. The Closing Years—a brief period of physical weakness and dependence on family or nursing care.

6. The Crowning Days—the days of dying—a period of only days, weeks, or months when we know that life is almost completed.

In this chapter we look at the closing years.

The main characteristic of the closing years is physical weakness and dependency, when it is no longer wise or practical to live alone, and where a move toward family care or nursing care is unavoidable. This final and irreversible giving up of certain as-

153

pects of independence, after probably sixty years of independence, takes time to get used to, but most older persons understand and welcome the change with gratitude and relief. For many years they have known the closing years were coming closer, and they are not surprised when these years arrive. Older persons remember caring for family and friends who went through the closing years, so they understand that in this time toward the end of old age, when weakness is increasing faster, it is beneficial and wise to accept the help of family or others. They adjust by suppressing their habits and attitudes of stubborn independence, accepting the change toward depending on others, while at the same time struggling to keep as much of their freedom, responsibilities, and roles as is practical.

The hardest part of giving up independence is usually the actual change of living arrangements: moving vans, papers to be signed, packing and unpacking. This is a time when tears and fears are certainly understandable, but when it is clear that the move is necessary, most older persons are surprised at how much easier the actual move was than they anticipated it would be.

Enemies of Independence: Weakness and Ill health

Look at this list of *physical weaknesses:*

1. Muscle weakness: leg muscles, ankle muscles, and back muscles. Even the act of standing and supporting one's own weight becomes more and more difficult. Sitting may even be a difficulty, and getting out of the bathtub or easy chairs is a strain.

2. Poor eyesight.

3. Poor hearing.

4. Weak heart and lungs: these two weaknesses often go together. It is not uncommon in the closing years for heart and lungs to have only 5 percent of their former maximum capacity, and 3 percent is not unusual. This makes a short walk or climbing a flight of stairs a strenuous workout.

5. Weak hand grip and weak feet.

6. Weak bladder.

7. Dizziness and poor sense of balance.

8. Brittle bones and stiff joints.

9. Any amount of overweight compounds other weaknesses. Any combinations of the above weaknesses can result in the decision to give up independence and accept the help of family or others.

Look at this list of *health problems, chronic illnesses, and diseases:*

1. Hypertension, due to many causes.

2. Atherosclerosis and arteriosclerosis, both of which reduce our physical working capacity.

3. Arthritis, causing chronic pain in the joints.

4. Emphysema and various lung ailments.

5. Broken limbs and dislocations.

6. Strokes and all forms of paralysis and handicaps.

This list could be much longer, but it is long enough to remind us of the full assortment of health problems that can lead us to the decision to give up independent living.

The enemies of independence are, then, physical weakness and ill health. We do not need to make the move to depending on others until we sense that it is no longer wise for us to live alone because we cannot care for ourselves properly. The decision is, of course, one that the older person must make, and family and physicians usually interfere only when they are of the opinion that the older person is procrastinating unwisely.

In the majority of instances, older persons have fairly good judgment about the proper time for the move to dependent living. Olive, age seventy-nine, had enjoyed her busy life and her own small house since her husband had died many years earlier. But when she had a slight stroke and was found unconscious on her kitchen floor, she did some serious thinking about her future and began to spend more and more time staying with her niece. She kept her little house and was still there several days a week, but her time at home was getting less and less as the niece pleaded with her not to live alone.

Then one day while Olive was puttering at home she fell and broke her arm, and it was several hours before she could be picked up and taken to hospital. This double negative—the broken arm and the hours before any help arrived—was enough to help Olive and the niece to work out the details of Olive's move away from independence to what became a long and mutually enjoyable period of living with the niece. This brief example illustrates the advantage of leaving the decision to the older person, even when there is high risk and danger from weakness and/or ill health. Olive enjoyed her closing years partly because she knew she had struggled to be independent, but she had proved to herself that independence was no longer possible.

Many older persons want the right to decide for themselves, and their decisions are usually better. Art surprised everyone when he came out of hospital at age eighty, after heart surgery, and lived alone enjoyably for nine more years before going to a nursing care home. (He preferred not to live with any of his devoted children!) Every life is unique and different, and Art knew his uniqueness and what would be best for him. When the time comes, each of us must look for very unique and personal solutions that will mean we can make the best of our closing years.

Living with Family or with Others: Which?

Here again, when there is a choice, the older person should make the choice. What are the alternatives, and what do most older persons choose?

1. Only 20 percent of those over age sixty-five are living alone; a full 80 percent of persons over age sixty-five are living with someone else.

2. Only 25 percent of those over age sixty-five are living with their adult children, but this percentage rises to 70 percent of all those over aged sixty-five who are living with their adult children in the last two years of life. Living with one's adult children is not a preferred living arrangement in North America and Western Europe, but older persons accept this arrangement for the closing years.

3. Seventy-five percent of the independent elderly live within twenty miles of one of their offspring, and 66 percent of the inde-

pendent elderly who have children see at least one of their children within a twenty-four-hour period. Old people don't like living with their offspring, but they like living close to them. As old people get weaker, they like to move closer to their offspring, even next door or down the street.

4. Fifty-five percent of those over age sixty are married and living together, and marriage and longevity go hand in hand. But by the closing years, the last two years of life, a large majority have lost their spouse.

5. Forty percent of childless older persons live with a brother, sister, or other relatives who assume the role responsibility of a son or daughter.

6. Only 2 percent of those age sixty-five to seventy-four are living in any kind of a nursing home.

7. Only 7.5 percent of those age seventy-five and up are living in any kind of institution.

8. Forty-eight percent of all admissions to places such as nursing homes are dead within three years.

9. Thirty percent of older persons spend their last year in a nursing home.

The two most important statistics in this section are: (a) Seventy percent of older persons spend their closing years with family or friends; (b) Thirty percent of older persons spend their last year in an institution.

Thus, the majority of older persons spend the closing years living with family or friends. In some of these instances the older person and family are very frustrated, and it is not the best arrangement. In still other instances, the arrangement is idyllic. In the majority of instances there are difficult adjustments for both the older person and the family, but the end result is worth the effort, and the elderly person and family or friends are pleased with the outcome.

Moving in with Family

If your relationship with your children in recent years has been marred by misunderstanding, unpleasantness, and unkindness, and if you have had difficulty in standing up for your rights, don't move in with family. If they were bad before, they may very well be worse now. If you have already moved in with family, and the arrangement is not hopeful, fight for your rights; and if you lose, then try to move out and move forward to something better. If family members are abusive, move out and do not return.

On the pleasant side of this topic, your family probably does want you very much. Give the new living arrangement your best effort. Scale down your expectations of each of the members of the family. Expect nothing from them, and you will never be disappointed. Have reasonable expectations of yourself and them, and it should work out better. A common problem is discovering that problems in a family that we thought had been dealt with have not really been solved, just hidden. Of course, when we move into a family setting, the tensions, conflicts, and immaturities can no longer be hidden, and we soon find out any sordid details. But imperfection and sin are universal, and we should be patient and forgiving about the family's problems. This will encourage the family to be patient with us when we have our very weak days.

Whatever you do, don't take sides with some family members in family disagreements, or you may be buying yourself a one-way ticket out of that family. Your responsibility is to be neutral in family arguments. In fact, absent is better than neutral, so if you are caught in the presence of an argument, just quietly excuse yourself from the room while letting both sides know that whatever they can agree on together is fine with you.

Be sure to have plenty of interests, activities, and responsibilities that are your very own. The previous two chapters apply very much to the closing years, so reread them from the point of view of living with family in the closing years.

Give the family a rest from you if opportunity comes for you to visit another family member or a friend.

Be sure to have time each day for privacy, as you need time for yourself.

Remember that when you live with someone else, their household rules apply to you. Go along with their rules, namely:

Daily shaving, bathing, change of clothes and bedding, hair cut, and hair styling;

Time for bed and getting up;

Habits—smoking, etc.

You may not like their rules, but the rules apply to you when you are living under their roof.

Caroline was age eighty-two when she moved in with her daughter and family. Caroline loved the family life after years of isolation, but she was very upset that her daughter's rules seemed so tough, and three rules seemed tougher than the rest:

Rule 1: Go to the hair stylist weekly. This was wasteful, Caroline thought. True, her hair was always beautiful now, and she received many compliments about it, but wouldn't once a month be enough? And what a money savings! (Caroline had plenty of savings after a lifetime of frugality.) The daughter wouldn't give an inch. So Caroline kept going.

Rule 2: A bath daily, along with clean undergarments and deodorants, and wearing only her best clothes every day of the week. Daughter was so helpful with the baths, and Caroline appreciated this, but why wear her best clothes? She should save these for some future events. "No way, Mom, you are going to look and smell your very best for every day you have left, and that's final." And the daughter even threw away some tattered and faded aprons, dresses, and slippers which made Caroline fume and pout for a day or two. But it was difficult to argue with her daughter when the grandchildren and their friends kept saying, "Gramma, you just look terrific!" and Caroline knew it was true!

Rule 3: "Mom, we expect you to come out to the living room for one full hour to visit whenever anyone drops over to the house for any reason." So Caroline had to leave her bedroom and hobble out to see the neighbors, the grandchildren, and the grandchildren's friends. Of course, Caroline was a sports fanatic and knew all the top NBA, NFL, and baseball teams, so how could she keep quiet when the younger ones were talking sports? How the younger ones loved to tease her when her favorite team was losing. Then too, the younger ones often enjoyed talking to Gramma about their boyfriend-girlfriend problems, and Caroline knew how to be a good listener with only an occasional insightful question and with only a minimal amount of giving advice. In fact, she usually stayed out in the living room or kitchen with the company for much more than the required hour, and the daughter was very pleased about this. "Mom, just remember, we can't afford to do many expensive things for you, but we do want you to be a part of all family activities and visits of our neighbors and friends." As Caroline got used to this rule, she wished she had thought of it for herself. Otherwise, she could have easily made excuses and withdrawn into a shell of self-pity. Then she would have been the loser!

One advantage of living with family is the maintenance of significant close relationships. Older persons suffer from isolation when they are separated from those for whom they feel the most affection and attachment, so living with family prevents this isolation. But family living does not prolong independence, as Caroline discovered through the three house rules of her daughter. These were the closing years, and she was depending on her family more and more as she slowly grew weaker.

Nursing Care Is Sometimes Better than Family Care

The negatives of nursing home care are known to everyone.

1. *Bureaucratic.* The institution may exist for its own rules and regulations and for its officers who enforce the rules. The residents get lost in the regulations. In such cases of bureacracy there can often be a form of dictatorship by the various subgroups in the institution:

a. Dictatorship of the housekeeping staff. This results in removal of pets, personal belongings, hobby material, food and "clutter" —all supposedly in the name of cleanliness, but in fact it's because the housekeeping staff is too lazy to allow cluttered bedrooms, as cleaning does take longer. Yet personal belongings, hobbies, "clutter," and pets are essential to provide an enriched life for nursing home residents. What a good thing that nursing care homes today are so much wiser and better on average than they were fifteen years ago. But still, there is no finer way to evaluate the suitability of a nursing care home than by inspecting the degree to which the housekeeping staff dictate a policy of emptiness and sterility by removal of personal belongings, hobbies, and pets.

b. Dictatorship of the kitchen and dietary staff. This results in a regimented plan of three heavy square meals a day, and never mind if this is not satisfactory for all patients.

Yet this is not in keeping with the needs of the elderly in the closing years. Why? First, it is well known that heavy meals require the body to draw a heavy supply of blood away from the brain. This results in sleepiness after heavy meals. Three bigger meals a day, as is the policy in poor quality nursing care homes, often results in three after-meal naps, which in turn result in sleeping pills to sleep fully through the night. Second, older persons do not flush sleeping pills efficiently from their system, so a pill taken the night before often results in sleepiness all through the morning. This morning sleepiness, added to sleepiness after heavy meals, often means the resident is sleeping most of his or her life away: all because the kitchen-dietary does not wish to provide nutritious light snacks more often and only one moderate-sized meal per day.

2. *Impersonal Aspects of Institutions.* Institutions sometimes remove choices and personal preferences to the degree that our sense of self is weakened. Whereas the institution should be on guard against "doing things for people," and instead should be pushing the residents to continue mastery of their environment and doing for themselves as much as possible for as long as possible, many institutions see the model resident as the one who is quiet, makes no demands of staff, and shows no initiative to keep going at as full a pace as possible. No wonder this depersonalized aspect frequently leads to depression because the residents do not know how to recover their sense of self-worth in the institutional regime. (The quiet negative!)

But in spite of these negative aspects of institutional care (Let's admit it: some nursing homes are ineffective, destructive, and demoralizing), institutions are sometimes better than families as a place to spend your closing years. What are the advantages of nursing care in a good nursing care home?

A. Family and friends can usually come to visit often without the extra burden of an invalid or semi-invalid parent or family member.

B. Nursing care is around the clock on a twenty-four-hour basis.

C. Some staff members are very loving and personal. They become the best friend an older person could ever hope for. They listen as personal fears and frustrations are shared. They listen as we reminisce about our lives. They advise and reassure as good friends should. They understand about our chronic pain or our feelings of uncertainty.

D. The best thing about nursing care is the new friends we can enjoy who are old like us. Older persons are happier, researchers tell us, when they can identify with their age group. Older persons need other older persons. They need contact with their peers. Kinship, comradeship, friendship, love, social activities, quiet dialogues—all of these beautiful things happen regularly when older persons enjoy life in a better nursing care home.

Look at these examples: Louise, age seventy-nine, came as a resident to a better nursing care home, and in three weeks she was starting to fall in love with fellow resident Jake, age seventy-six. That love affair purred and then sputtered off and on for years, to the delight of both.

John, always a great talker, came to a nursing care home from thirty years of living alone on the farm, and though he was eighty, it only took him six months to make the best friend he ever had in his fellow resident engineer buddy Bob, age seventy-eight.

Emory, age eighty-four, hated leaving his house and his garden, but he found a much better life in a better nursing care home because of the kinship with others of his own ethnic persuasion.

Shirley loved the religious and fellowship emphasis in her Mennonite personal care facility. Saint Joseph's residence met the needs of Pearl and many elderly Polish residents who could not speak a word of English though they had all lived fifty years in a very large western city. All of these persons found new life and excitement in their closing years because of the attitudes, atmosphere, and activity of a better nursing care facility.

It is very possible to get into the wrong nursing home—one that is not suited to a particular person's needs. It then becomes an urgent matter to *get out of that home* and into the right home. This is easier said than done, but it is not impossible.

Tom worked hard to find the right spot for his elderly father and was pleased with the results when father settled very well into a different home.

Ellen couldn't understand her mother's complaints, but Mother was obviously happy in the next nursing home that was found.

Another relevant point is how to maintain motivation in older institutionalized adults. A number of points are relevant, from a major study by Filer and O'Connell:

(a) Residents should manage their own medications.

(b) Residents should have full responsibility for keeping appointments dependably.

(c) Residents should participate in some productive, constructive work.

(d) Residents should be responsible for housekeeping in their own living area.

(e) Residents should be responsible for their own personal appearance and hygiene.

(f) Personal laundry is a responsibility of residents.

(g) Finances should be managed on their own.

(h) Residents should be held responsible for their behavior.

Residents may ask for help in any of the above areas, but it should still be their responsibility.

Senility Is Not for You

Not too many years ago scientific research established that old brains are usually as good as young brains, and sometimes old brains are better. We have looked at this scientific research in detail (chap. 4). Do you remember the highlights? See if these points ring the bells of your memory:

1. Active brains maintain their full capability. It is mental

exercise that maintains mental ability at full strength, while mental inactivity results in slow and ineffective mental functioning. Old brains need regular mental work: things to learn, problems to solve, and memory to be exercised. Think, reason, argue, debate, plan, memorize, create, read, study—and you will be giving your brain its best opportunity to be as clear as a bell and in top shape at age ninety-nine.

2. Medical problems—especially hypertension, circulatory disorders, fevers, and infections—cause the brain to slow down and function poorly, but proper successful treatment of medical problems restores full brain potential quickly in most cases.

3. Depression, anxiety, boredom, and loneliness—the four negatives that often bring about positive consequences—signal the need for some constructive action and meaningful life changes. When these four negatives are worked through successfully, then the brain usually functions effectively again.

4. Our brains do wear out and slow down, but in the majority of instances age is less important than activity level in predicting how much older persons know and how well they can reason and remember. So get your old brain busy again, starting gradually and over time building up a "full head" of steam.

One minor point should be mentioned about memory. Many older people get frustrated when their "train of thought runs off the track." Some can remember what color of dress they wore to a party fifty years ago but not what they had for breakfast.

Some people forget, if they wait for a break in the conversation, so have come to the habit of "butting in" by saying, "I'm sorry, but if I don't mention this right now, I'll forget it." This is fine as it is more frustrating for an older person to lose a thought and try to remember it than to interject a comment into a conversation.

Family and nursing personnel should realize this and accept it.

High-Risk Living—Challenge Yourself

The closing years are the best time for high-risk living, in which we risk possible failure and embarrassment in personal, emotional, and social areas.

What kinds of risk should be taken, and what are the possible big advantages to be gained?

1. *Risk rejection.* Be the first person to say hello, even if the other person ignores you. Be friendly, and when others fail to respond, that is their problem. Whatever you offer of your mind, heart, skills, intentions, and person, others may refuse; but if you would like to offer, take the high risk of rejection anyway and approach them. Offer to write a letter, offer to read a story, offer to listen, and offer to be a friend. But offering yourself is not enough—asking is part of risking rejection. Ask someone to sit and talk. Ask someone for help. Even if you are afraid, ask anyway.

2. *Risk injury*—not ignorantly, but as a well-calculated risk. When we have had a tumble before, and when the weather is icy and wet, we may still want to go to a hockey game. If we are asked to go, under responsible terms, we should say yes, even though there is a very small risk of falling or slipping or getting bruised and shaken up. Over the many years of a long life you have gotten wise enough to know where the dangers are, but don't stop living because there are dangers in a variety of places.

3. *Risk failure.* You will never fail if you never try. What are some things you would like to try to do? How about knitting or growing tomatoes or making supper or teaching a lesson or helping a friend? Is failure so terrible that we shouldn't even try?

Older persons need to challenge themselves every day. The challenge is to make today significant and meaningful in terms of everything we believe is good and true. As time is running out, it becomes more important to make the most of each day. As we become weaker, we must try harder and more wisely. Life is always a risk, but in the closing years the high risk of living is the stimulation we need to make us want to live better.

Do not imagine that it is ever too late to start or to start again. Grandma Moses didn't start to paint until she was over eighty, and actor George Burns still does movies, commercials, and guest appearances at a very old age.

Enrich the Bedroom—It Is Your Home Base

Our world is shrinking in the closing years, and in many cases the bedroom becomes the focal point of life. So enrich the bedroom. First of all, if it is a large room, all the better, to allow for comfortable sitting chairs, tables, TV, dressers, aquarium, plants, canary, and books.

It should be inviting to others. People will come to visit more often if there is a place to sit. It should be inviting to children— games and puzzles for them, a cookie jar or candy jar. What better way to have grandchildren want to come for further visits than to consider their needs too? Photograph albums are an essential, as a focus for one's friends and one's family. Current issues of magazines are good to have.

The bedroom of the closing years should contain some of life's greatest treasures: family Bible, old clock, treasured furniture, wall pictures, awards and trophies, historic portraits, and family pictures.

The bedroom should focus on activities, including hobbies, projects, chess game, plants, pets, and leisure reading.

The bedroom should double as a classroom for self-education because we should be learning and studying as long as we live. Books, study courses, and writing materials are all helpful.

Television in the bedroom is very good for the news, sports, dramas, education, and other features a person may enjoy.

Reminisce Together

To reminisce is to recall and to relate one's past, and this process is invaluable for the person in the closing years. Why?

(1) Reminiscing activates memory, and active memories stay at full strength and even improve. Irma, age eighty-six, says to Anna, age eighty-four, "Anna, where did you go to school in grade one?" Anna replies, "That was in the convent in the south of Munich just a few years before World War I." Then Irma and Anna share memories, and their facial muscles are animated

beautifully, their eyes sparkle, and their voices are rich in expressiveness as they share personal memories and work at becoming better friends.

(2) Reminiscing leads to satisfying activities and social experiences. At Red River Personal Care Home, some enjoyable reminiscing about "food our mothers used to make" led to a tease about fathers and males being poor cooks. One tease led to another, and the result was a special social baking event in which five of the male residents each baked one loaf of homemade bread, with each inexperienced male baker receiving guidance and direction from an experienced female baker-teacher. The residence activities worker creatively turned this event into a highlight of the season, as the bread was judged in a contest, with everyone having plenty of laughs.

(3) Fond memories should be treasured and shared. The great events of the past should not be forgotten. Horrors of our past sometimes haunt us, and these horrors can be crowded into a corner if there are pleasant memories to share with others. Some of us have been overexposed to Grandpa's favorite story of his youth, so we will not overtell our favorite story. But it is an even greater error not to share our past at all.

(4) Read this prayer of a seventeenth-century nun (1659 AD!).

Growing Old

Lord, Thou knowest better than I know myself that I am growing older and will someday be old.

Keep my mind free from the recital of endless details; give me wings to get the point. Seal my lips on my aches and pains. They are increasing, and love of rehearsing them is becoming sweeter as the years go by. I dare not ask for grace enough to enjoy the tales of others' pains, but help me to endure them with patience.

Keep me from the fatal habit of thinking I must say something on every subject and on every occasion. Release me from craving to straighten out everybody's affairs. Make me thoughtful but not moody, helpful but not bossy. With my vast store of wisdom, it seems a pity not to use it all, but Thou knowest, Lord, that I want a few friends at the end.

12

The Crowning Days—
A Study of Dying

Pennies on the Eyes of the Living

For almost one hundred years Western society has not wanted to face the facts of dying and death. The reason has been our focus on improving and extending life. The twentieth century has been a wonder age with cures for disease, medicines to keep us healthy, vitamins for every problem, and fresh reports every year that people are living longer and longer. During this great focus on life, dying was ignored and shunned, and people would not say the word *death* if they could avoid it. "He passed on," they would say. Or, "He is no longer with us." We had taken the penny off the dead man's eyes, and we had placed that death penny on the eyes of the living, so the living would not have to face the facts of dying and death.

Now the pendulum which avoided death has swung the other way, and death and dying have become a sociomedical fad of the eighties. Before, we would not think about dying; now we dwell on it. Every week there is a new seminar on dying, led by an "expert" who has considered the subject in depth for at least six weeks and who, himself or herself, took a course on the subject and got a certificate. TV commercials now compare cremation and burial costs and try to sell first one and then the other approach. Prearranged plots, the question of whether we should tell dying persons they are dying, withdrawal of life-support systems from the dying,

169

rights of the dying, stages of dying—all these topics are considered in the weekend section of the newspaper and in parlor talk. Lobby groups are pressuring legislators to change the laws to assist, protect, and guide the dying. The dead man's pennies on the eyes of the living have been taken off, and we now consider the whole subject of dying and death with more knowledge and more compassion.

Now that a majority of us do have our eyes open because of the current fascination with dying and death, what remains of importance to be said about dying as the conclusion of a better half of life? Let us list the points of importance, and then discuss each of them in detail:

1. God is in control of our living and dying and death. "The Lord gives and the Lord takes away" (Job 1:21).

2. Sudden death is the usual way to die.

3. Dying sometimes means fading away.

4. Who will walk to the edge with me? The importance of companions for the dying.

5. Don't feel guilty if you are afraid! Four *good* reasons to be afraid of dying.

6. Dying is a time of crowning.

7. The resurrection and the life.

Let us look together at each of these aspects of dying, remembering that dying is part of living, and dying ought to be a fitting conclusion and summation of the better half of life.

The Lord Gives and the Lord Takes Away

When shall I die? How shall I die? Shall I suddenly drop dead, or shall I fade away due to weakness or disease? The answers to these questions are unknown except to God Himself, and He rarely reveals the time or circumstances. All we can know is that God decides, according to His own holy purpose and will, the day of our birth, the place of our birth, and the circumstances of our birth. "*The Lord Gives*" . . . He gives life according to His own secret providence. Next, He sustains, protects, and directs each life, again according to His own counsel. *He numbers our days* and years according to our allotment of time, determined in length by His decision (see Ps. 90:10-12). Finally, *He "takes away"* our life when we arrive at that appointed day and hour. The manner of His taking away of our life is also predetermined by His own immutable judgment. In summary, God decides the day of our birth, He decides the length of our life, and He decides the date and circumstances of our death. He does not promise us an easy death, but He does promise to be there with us in the days or hours or minutes of our dying.

God is sovereign over all of life and death. Life begins, prospers, fades, and ends—all according to the word and wisdom of the sovereign Lord of all. My responsibility is to care for my body, nurture my life, and seek to fulfill my life, but He will decide when my hour has come. Just as I have learned to depend upon Him in the living of my life, so I must also learn to depend on Him in my dying and death. "The Lord takes away . . . blessed be the name of the Lord." In other words: "Thank You, Lord, that the day of my death is not decided by accident, chance, bad luck, magic, Satan, or any other factor. Your wisdom has decided the day of my death, and because your wisdom has decided the day, it is therefore the perfect day for me to die. Bless the Lord for His decision."

Do not question God's decision about the time and circumstances of your dying and death. You will get nowhere if you question Him. Accept His decision. Two apostles were thrown in prison: Peter was released from prison, but the apostle James was beheaded. This was God's sovereign decision about which one lived, not the tetrarch's decision. John the Baptist was also beheaded in prison at the request of a dancing girl! Imagine John the Baptist—God's faithful servant, full of the Holy Spirit from birth—preaching and preparing the way of the Lord: devoted, spiritual, obedient, and only desiring to serve his God. God had decided the date and circumstances of John the Baptist's death, and God was with John the Baptist in his dying. The Lord took away John the Baptist's life, not the dancing girl, and we must learn to accept God's sovereignty over all of life and death.

Stop worrying about the date and circumstances of your dying and death. This is all in God's hands. Leave it to Him. Praise Him that He knows better than you, and the decision is in His hand. Make your preparations to die, and leave the timing up to Him.

Sudden Death Is the Usual Way to Die

Many people experience death suddenly. They are alive and busy, pursuing life in all its complexity and intrigue, and with little or no warning they drop dead. Is this sudden death the preferred way to die? Some say yes, some say no, but the answers are irrelevant because we have no choice or say in the matter. Preferred or not preferred as a manner of dying, sudden death is the way of the majority of humans. Helen, age sixty-three, was in the kitchen at 4:30 PM getting supper when she suddenly felt a shortness of breath. She called her doctor, and then she drove over to the hospital one mile away. She walked into Emergency; her doctor met her and asked her to lay down and take oxygen. In five more minutes she slipped into unconsciousness, and she died before 5:00 PM. The time from her first symptom to her death was less than thirty minutes. How many of our friends have died suddenly in old age or in youth! Bob, age thirty-five, in what seemed to be perfect health, died in his sleep. Fran, age forty-four, had a nap after lunch and died in her sleep. Dave, age sixty-one, died instantly after his morning shave. Kelly, age seventy, was having coffee with a kitchen full of friends when she died instantly.

Look at the following percentages of causes of death at various ages in two major categories: cancer and heart-related deaths. Cancer is the cause of death in 11.3 percent of all deaths, while heart attacks and strokes account for 73.5 percent of all deaths. In the age grouping sixty-five to seventy-four, take note that cancer is the cause of 7.93 percent of deaths, while heart attacks and strokes account for 77 percent of deaths. In the age grouping seventy-five to eighty-four, cancer is the cause of 10.9 percent of deaths, while heart attacks and strokes account for 70 percent of deaths. In the age grouping eighty-five+ note that cancer is the cause of 4.3 percent of deaths, while heart attacks and strokes account for 76 percent of deaths.

The statistics about the cause of death indicate that the majority of us are going to die suddenly or with only a brief warning. In an effort to provide guidelines and rules for living the second half of life in a better way, what guidelines can be given to this large group who die suddenly? There is no special advice possible except the following:

1. You will probably die suddenly without warning, so, in addition to keeping the other rules, keep yourself in a state of readiness to die, even in the midst of the hussle and bussle of your life. Is your will made out? Is your life insurance in order? Are your personal papers organized and available to your executor and trustee? Have you instructed your executor about your commitments and intentions?

2. What personal sharing do you need to do with spouse, family, friends, and business associates? Do it now, even if it should turn out that you live another twenty-five years.

3. Live every day in a state of readiness to meet your Maker, for you know not what hour you will have to surrender your life.

Dying Sometimes Means Fading Away

Dying sometimes means fading away. In such instances we get weaker and weaker as one or another vital system fails us. We notice our increasing weakness or steady loss of weight, and we make estimates of how much time remains. René had very little pain because the hospital followed a policy of painless dying. But she watched her weight as it plunged to one hundred pounds, then ninety pounds, then eighty pounds. Not that her weight was a preoccupation, but she used her weight as a rough gauge to estimate the month of her death. Later, she did not have the strength to walk around, so she remained in her bed resting comfortably on an inflatable cushion. The next stage was the tiredness, the hard work of breathing, the impossible task of chewing, swallowing, excreting, and the exhaustion of bathing, combined with the delicious sips of tea through a strawlike tube. In the final stage

Age-Specific Death Rates per 100,000 Population per Year by Cause

Cause of Death	All Ages	65-74	74-85	85+
Neoplasm, stomach (cancer)	12	67	123	156
Neoplasm, colon	16	87	167	220
Neoplasm, lung	22	123	105	74
Neoplasm, breast	14	55	82	135
Neoplasm, prostate	7	45	116	171
Diabetes mellitus	16	96	167	174
Subarachnoid and cerebral thrombosis	60	261	749	1,686
Cerebral embolism and thrombosis	32	152	517	1,341
Other CNS vascular diseases	8	34	137	449
Arteriosclerotic heart disease	278	1,433	1,306	6,878
Endocarditis and myocardial degeneration	29	118	438	1,465
Other heart disease	11	47	116	277
Hypertensive heart disease	35	179	446	933
Other hypertensive diseases	7	26	81	221
General arteriosclerosis	18	56	300	1,394
Chronic and unspecified nephritis	6	21	45	101
Influenza and pneumonia	32	102	316	999
Emphysema	5	33	43	46
Senility, ill defined	7	22	49	183
Accidents, falls	11	33	137	513

there was a little more waiting, a great deal of sleeping, and at last the long rest began.

These are the common physical stages of dying as experienced by René and by countless others:

1. Increasing weakness and confinement to bed.
2. Exhaustion even from breathing, chewing, swallowing, and excreting.
3. Much more sleeping and periods of unconsciousness.
4. Unconsciousness.
5. Death.

In our modern age of effective pain relief, there is very little pain in dying. Doctors calculate the increasing amount of pain relief that will be required, and the dying person receives relief before experiencing the need. Dying is thus a comfortable experience for most persons, and so it ought to be.

The experience of dying is usually unique and individual. René's experience was not Jack's because Jack had a different set of weaknesses: thirst, confused thinking, poor vision, and fatigue. As his wife Sarah sat beside Jack, she had to help him remember he had just had some juice, even though it didn't seem to quench his insatiable thirst. In the last three days Jack was no longer conscious. The doctor assured Sarah that Jack was not in pain and would not wake up again. The doctor turned out to be right.

The physical symptoms of dying are a clue to doctors and loved ones, who use the clue to give their dying friend as much comfort as possible. And some day in the future, when the comforter's turn comes to die, that is all he or she will desire in return.

Who Will Go to the Edge with Me?

We have looked at the physical aspects of dying, but the emotional aspects of dying are also important.

Lillian, age seventy-eight, went for tests; when the doctor gave her the test results, she had four months to live, give or take a few weeks. The next ten days were filled with a great mixture of feelings: first a wave of *anger*, followed by *sadness*, then a wave of *fear*. She even found herself *denying* her problem and pretending she was healthy. Then followed a week of serious reassessment, based on *accepting* her situation and calculating how to get the most out of the time she had remaining. Then came peace of mind, with only occasional regrets and fears. She did live another four months, and those four months were the finest display of her virtue and wisdom that her family had ever seen. Four months of dying is a lot of dying, but Lillian did it well.

It was different for Ed, who was ninety-four. No doctor came with pronouncements. Ed and his family just knew his heart was getting weaker and weaker. He simply got to the place where standing up was more than he could manage. Then sitting became too much. Finally raising a hand, thinking, smiling, and talking—all of those activities were too much, and Ed died—at home, without fear but with friends and family around him. The way it happened was simple: his wife was sitting in a chair beside his bed doing her knitting and talking to him. It occurred to her that Ed looked sweaty, and she got up and shouted loudly (his hearing always had been poor), "Ed, would you like me to take off one blanket? How about a face wash?" As he could not speak and seemed unable to make himself clear to her, she pulled one blanket down halfway, then walked to the washroom for a damp facecloth. In those few seconds—perhaps forty seconds—Ed's heart stopped, and he died. What his emotions were at the end is difficult to say: probably fatigue, some boredom, a little confusion, but gratitude for his wife and the familiar surroundings of home.

Jean, age seventy-one, had to die in the hospital. She required life-support systems which could extend her life for several months. As she and her husband Chris talked about dying, she shared with him a concern of most, but not all, persons who are about to die. Her concern? That she should not die alone or among strangers. She wanted someone there at the very end to hold her hand in her last hours. She wanted to know, "Who will go to the edge with me?" Her husband listened and looked at this woman who was the great love of his life, and said, "Jean, I promise you that I will be with you to the end." That is just how the end came for Jean—with Jean and Chris holding hands in her hospital room.

Are you prepared to spend time with the dying? Are you willing to go to the edge with a friend or family member? Will you hold a hand until the end?

Do Not Feel Guilty Because You Are Afraid

The Christian views death as a deliverance and a promotion. "To me life is Christ, and death gain; . . . What I should like is to depart and be with Christ; that is better by far" (Phil. 1:21-24).

Death is therefore something to be desired when the time comes, and it makes no sense for the Christian to be afraid of death.

To be afraid of dying is a different matter. Dying is the prelude to death, and dying may last a few moments or a few months. Four elements of dying are often associated with *fear*. When these elements are involved, we as Christians should *not* feel guilty or ashamed that we are afraid of dying.

1. *The fear of pain and discomfort.* The possibility of a painful dying can cause fear, and this fear should motivate us to seek pain relief as required. Do not feel guilty of the fear of a painful dying. Be prepared to ask for pain relief.

2. *The fear for the future of one's family, congregation, and ideals.* Mary, age sixty-eight, was dying in the hospital, surrounded by family and friends, including her retarded forty-year-old son. She feared for the future of her son, but she gained a sense of relief as she realized she had done what she could to prepare her son for his future. It was all in God's hands, and she could leave it with Him.

3. *The fear of the unknown.* Herb did not know if he would linger in semiconsciousness near the end, and this unknown made him afraid. His uncle had died the year before, and Herb had watched him alternate between confused semiconsciousness and unconsciousness. Now Herb wished that he might not put his family through a similar prolonged dying. Herb also wondered, "How shall I die? By choking, by weakness and fatigue, or by a

sudden stopping of the heart?" He feared this unknown, and yet he knew the decision was not his to decide. He was able to leave the matter in the hands of Him for whom there is no unknown.

4. *The fear of embarrassment.* Some of the dying are afraid that in their confusion and weakness they may be indiscreet and thus cause their family shame and embarrassment.

From these four elements we see that there are often legitimate reasons for the dying to be afraid. Let us learn to be sensitive as we comfort the dying, and this sensitivity should include an awareness and acceptance of their legitimate fears. They may wish to discuss these fears, in which case we should listen and respond with understanding.

The Resurrection and the Life

What is death? Death is a new beginning. Death is the first step in eternity. We put our hands into the hand of God, and without looking back, we take the big step. Good-bye earth, Hello Great Day!

On this earth we tasted life in miniature. This life was just a trial run to get us started in the right direction. Our threescore and ten years are just a very small sample of the great Day that begins at the instant of death.

In our own personal deaths we identify briefly with the death of Christ our Lord, who died for us. As quickly as we are dead, we then participate in His resurrection too, and the new life begins.

Jesus said, "I am the resurrection and I am life. If a man has faith in me, even though he die, he shall come to life" (John 11:25).

Jesus also said, "Set your troubled hearts at rest. Trust in God always; trust also in me. There are many dwelling-places [over there] in my Father's house; . . . I am going there on purpose to prepare a place for you. . . . I shall come again and receive you to myself, so that where I am you may be also; . . . I am the way; I am the truth and I am life; no one comes to the Father except by me" (John 14:1-6).

In dying we are letting go of this life, and we are preparing to meet our Maker. In death we meet Him face to face. In the new life we love Him; we walk with Him; in joy and excitement we serve Him and reign with Him forever and forever. So be it!

A Crowning Time

The dying should be honored in any and all ways that are appropriate. Ross had been a wise and loving spouse, parent, employer, deacon, and Christian friend. While he still had some energy and a sparkle in his eye—though that eye was nearly blind—and though Ross was bedridden and very weak, his family, congregation, and friends came daily and paid their respects and affection in an ongoing spirit of celebration. Ross blushed and smiled quite a few times as he listened to the praise of all those who came to visit and who sensed the great value of this life that was ebbing away. He was a great teaser in a gentle way; he listened to this praise and turned to his wife and joked, "You see, Ulna, I've been telling you all these years what a great guy I am. How come I'm just ordinary Ross in your books?" And Ulna looked lovingly at this man who was the great love of her life and teased back at him, "Because I know the truth about you, Ross, that is why!" In the last three weeks of fading strength and drifting consciousness, Ross reminisced, gave a few farewell instructions, and paid his own respects to the others. In the last two days he suddenly slipped into unconsciousness and never did awaken.

Crowning is, of course, for kings and heroes, but some of the dying should be crowned as well in order to recognize the highlights of a completed life and to remind the dying of our view of the true worth of their accomplishments. Crowning means several things:

1. *Crowning means thank you.* Thank you is of no value to the dead; but to the dying, thank you brings a sense of fulfillment that gives the readiness to let go of life when the time comes. Thank you should be expressed whenever there is the occasion to say it, but dying is a time for repeating all past thank yous. Norman made it back home to share in his old father's dying. "Dad, let me start from the beginning and repeat my thanks for everything.

Thanks for coaching me in baseball that time I was eight years old. That baseball season will always stand out in my memory because you were so encouraging to me. Thanks too for being so good to Mom over all the years. Thanks for helping Mary and me when we were first married, and thanks for being such a great grandparent. Thanks most of all for sharing your Christian faith with me and pointing me in the direction of a Spirit-filled life. And thanks for never giving up on me when I had those ignorant years when I was seventeen and eighteen." Dying should be a time of thanksgiving, when we express our thanks while there is still time.

2. *Crowning means a commitment.* Marilyn said to her dying mother, "Mom, besides all of those thank yous, I want you also to know that you have done a wonderful job with Jesse and Dad. We want to promise you that we will finish the work you started, and we will look after Jesse and Dad. How it will all work out I don't know, but you need have no worries about them because whatever they need, I will be there to help. If Dad should get drinking again, I will be there everyday until Jesse is fully grown. So relax and have no fear about that." After mother's death, Marilyn kept her word and her commitment, and she willingly did what she had to do for Jesse and Dad. It did all work out better than Marilyn and Mom could have wished.

3. *Crowning means comfort.* This is the medical age of painless dying. But some do not wish pain relief because of the dulled senses that accompany certain medications. In such cases it is valuable to reassure the dying that sleep and rest are important, and pain relief is important too for those who want to remember the dead in terms of comfort, not agony or pain. Aunt Helen came to the stage in her dying where regular morphine was necessary for her pain. Her niece Maureen and other family took Helen home from the hospital and kept her completely comfortable in her last two weeks, even though this meant that Aunt Helen was only awake and alert three or four hours per day. What a gracious way of honoring the dying!

4. *Crowning means companionship at the end.* Crowning in-

volves the honor of sharing the last days, hours, and moments. Go all the way to the edge with this dying person who went as far with you as he or she was able to go.

It is important to us, as the survivors, to say all of our thank-yous to the dying, whether we "feel" like saying these or not. If we know these thankyous ought to be said, we should go ahead and do our duty. Otherwise we may regret our silence afterward. Perry was a case in point. He knew he should have expressed his appreciation but didn't do so. "Well, there always seemed to be people around, and I was embarassed to speak up. Now, I wish I had sent a thank you to Mom or else blurted it out. Why did I let my shyness and inhibition hold me back?"

13

Growing Older Joyfully!

The Second Half of Life Is Better!

Let us review very briefly the highlights that have accentuated our study of the life span and the aging process. First, attitude is everything. A positive attitude can carry us through countless disasters. A negative attitude dwells on problems and misses all the opportunities.

Do you need an attitude overhaul to help you enjoy all the years ahead? The second half of life will have its share of frustrations and disappointments, but you should have learned by now that *attitude* goes a long way toward making the sky a beautiful blue.

To overhaul your attitude, get a number of truths firmly set in your mind:

1. Nobody owes you anything. It is up to you to make your life what you want it to be. Stop blaming others. Stop depending on them for so much.

2. Middle age and old age—all the years after thirty-five—are filled with excitements and adventures to be enjoyed. Don't spend even one moment in self-pity, wishing your life could have been different. Make some big changes if you need to, and get on with the business of living enthusiastically.

3. God has reconciled you to Himself through Jesus Christ. This exciting, encouraging truth is the basis of a positive attitude. You

are reconciled! Nothing else is so important. So celebrate your reconciliation through all your remaining years.

In the second half of your life, seek to share your wisdom with those who need it. Be friendly, humble, accessible, patient, radiant in faith, and share your wisdom with discretion and judgment. The second half of life is better when we focus on sharing our wisdom.

How to Find Real Joy in the Second Half of Life

Science says we should keep mentally and physically active as we get older. We should find new roles and new responsibilities each year to replace those which have ceased or faded away. This is all good advice.

The Christian view has much to add to science. True and lasting joy begins with awareness of God's great *love* for us as revealed through His Son Jesus Christ. If we want joy, we must respond to God's love and grace. The second half of life is much better when we use time to reexamine and strengthen the foundation of our faith.

If you want joy, do not pursue it! Instead, if you want joy, pursue virtue, and then with virtue comes joy.

If you want joy, pursue wisdom and noble adventures. There are things to do, while there is yet time, which have eternal consequences. Pursue the great things of life concerning meaning, purpose, values, and truth. The Christian strategy of joy is to invest your life in the service of Him from whom all blessings flow. Lose your life in His great cause, and joy will be a reward.

A Longer, Healthier, Better Half of Life

Seek to care for and fulfill your life by following the laws of health and longevity:
1. Be positive and hopeful about your future.
2. Be active—physically, mentally, emotionally, socially, and spiritually.
3. Break bad habits if you want to live a long and enjoyable life. Bad habits include: alcohol abuse, tobacco abuse, physi-

cal inactivity, marijuana and drug abuse, overweight, overwork, frequent exhaustion, and worry.

4. Prevent disease by fighting its causes and accepting medical treatment.
5. Eat properly.
6. Keep working.
7. Exercise if necessary.
8. Rest as required.
9. Relax in two ways:
   —by reducing anxiety.
   —by reducing muscle tension.

The Christian follows a disciplined approach to care of the body, preferring to do what one knows to be the best for the body without letting feelings and emotions dictate how one shall live.

Old Brains Are Better

Let us dump the youth cult, and let us get back to wisdom, in which we reverence and respect our premium citizens, the middle aged and the elderly, who alone can give the guidance and direction to create a better life and a better world.

Congregation and denominational leaders must recognize that older persons know more and are wiser. A new attitude must be expressed which honors our mothers, our fathers, our elders, and our citizens who are living in the second half of life.

Three Distinct Stages of Adulthood

Middle age starts at forty and ends at sixty.

Old age starts at sixty and usually lasts a long time!

These two age groupings should be used as a basis of Christian ministry. Congregations must minister to those in middle age who have the unique responsibilities and tasks we have already discussed in detail. This age group provides the leadership and energy to take the congregation forward in meaningful ministry.

Congregations must also minister to the elderly if they would hope to benefit from what the elderly can share, namely, wisdom.

The world is in desperate need of congregations which function as a unique cooperation between generations. All age groupings should minister and be ministered to in a New Testament congregation, and each generation should enrich and be enriched by the other generations.

This noble congregational goal of intergenerational cooperation is only achieved if we respond to the uniqueness and needs of each generation.

Mid-Life Crisis—The Road to the Better Half!

Youth does not last long, and sometime in the late thirties we begin to sense that youth is fading fast. This is the "noon" of life, and we begin to see youth for what it is, and we decide to let it go. This decision is not an easy one, and we often have regrets and misgivings, followed by renewed interest in and focus on the opportunities and challenges ahead.

If Christ is our way of confronting the aging process, and He is our basis of understanding the life span, the mid-life crisis is smoother and less turbulent. But even Christians sometimes need to be shaken out of their lethargy, so they will reassess their total situation and adjust to the changing pattern of strengths and weaknesses that will be experienced in the years ahead.

Males find the halfway point of life more difficult, but they come out of the self-evaluation process of mid-life ready to be more productive.

Mid-life consists primarily of a search for answers to questions about purpose, meaning, identity, and aging. Death and dying are also of concern. A successful mid-life crisis paves the way to a satisfying middle age: the years from forty-five to sixty-five.

The Productive Years—Age 45 to 55

This decade is the calm after the mid-life storm. We reach full adulthood at last, and this means we have a reasonably accurate assessment of our own strengths and weaknesses. We accept the fact of the inevitability of physical decline and increasing weakness, while at the same time reveling in our better judgment and discretion.

Are we mature? Maturity of mind is the essence of this period. We are self-aware, realistic in most instances, more rational, and less anxious, having a balance and perspective that cause the projects and tasks of our life to prosper.

Are we productive? Yes, because of our maturity. With less energy, we get more accomplished because of our maturity.

At times, in these years, we are caught in the "generation" squeeze because we are at that age when we are still supporting our offspring, and we are beginning to carry the weight of care of aging parents.

But more pleasant times are coming as we learn to break the parenting habit and enjoy the empty nest. This is also a time to revive the marital bond.

The Happy Time—Ages 55 to 65

Most persons, looking back on their years, note this decade—age fifty-five to sixty-five—as the happy time. But whatever is the happiest time, happiness is never an accident. Happiness comes from successful pursuit of a number of important goals:

A. *Wisdom,* in which we finally achieve that common sense and good judgment in living. The various elements of living—marriage, family, employment, social relationships, and responsibilities—are finally providing us with satisfaction. We sense that we are getting the different strands of endeavor together in a pattern of harmony based on wisdom.

B. *Virtue* also brings life satisfaction. We know we are doing our duty, acting responsibly, exercising self-control and kindness. We can live at peace with ourselves because of a good heart.

C. *Meaningful relationships* enrich our lives because we know how to manage our emotions and feelings in love, friendship, and acquaintance.

D. *Noble adventures* are the icing on the cake. Those who are involved in exciting and worthwhile projects have an extra source of satisfaction to enrich these happy years.

If any of these sources of life satisfaction are missing or absent, it becomes important to pursue the missing part. It is never too late to begin this pursuit because our rich experiences of life help us to make major progress quickly in the weaker area.

Growing Older—Age 65 and Up!

A number of dismal facts of old age are really opportunities if we have a positive outlook. Friends moving away, friends dying, our own ill health—each of these dismal facts can be a spur to seek out new friends or pursue health with reasonable care if we can take our eyes off the problem and see the opportunities around us.

You may at age sixty-five have another twenty-five years of living ahead of you. What are you going to do with all of this time? Will you see the exciting, encouraging, unlimited possibilities ahead? Or will you dwell on negatives?

Begin your old age by making whatever decisions you need to make that will keep you going forward.

You should:

—Share your wisdom, or miss the point of old age.

—Use your body and brain, or watch them wither away from disuse.

—Learn to roll with the punches. As life deals you a rough punch to the chin—or to your pocketbook or to your social life—learn to soften the blow and to recover quickly.

—Enjoy your peers: the other elderly.

Growing old is whatever you make of it. Why not decide now to get a reputation for a positive outlook based on a focus on God's goodness? Count your blessings and enjoy the years ahead.

Growing Older with a Positive Outlook!

We are responsible for our character and personality. The life span is an ongoing endeavor to create a character that will serve us well. We ought to be continually trying to improve and upgrade our character and personality.

Self-esteem, the basis of a positive outlook, comes from looking at our character and being pleased with what we see, even if we are still trying to improve in some areas.

The mind has four negative strategies which are aimed at character growth and improvement. These four adaptive life-serving strategies are:

1. Depression, which always aims at improvement in character and life situation.

2. Anxiety, which motivates us to make changes in our thinking, behavior, and life situation.

3. Loneliness, which pressures us to improve our social strategy.

4. Boredom, which motivates us to get on with the pursuit of what we really want.

These four negative strategies are self-improvements in disguise. If we learn to work successfully with these four negatives, we will have made major progress toward a positive outlook.

Have you learned how to make depression work for you? Learn how to make all four negatives work for you.

The Closing Years

The time finally comes—unless we die suddenly—when we must give up our independence, and we must move in with family or others. The enemies of independence, which force the move, are physical weakness and/or ill health. For safety and health reasons we must no longer live alone, and the question comes: If I have a choice, should I move in with family, or should I opt for nursing care? Seventy percent spend their final year with family while 30 percent move to a nursing home. It is important to remember that family is the right move for some, and it is a very wrong move for others. Do not be sentimental when you make this decision. If you have not had pleasant experiences with family in recent years, talk about the move in detail *before* you move in. Many are much happier in nursing care because the activities and fellowship can be excellent in the better nursing care facilities.

Learn to take risks in the closing years. Be friendly even at the risk of rejection. Be active, with discretion, even at the risk of injury. Try new activities, even at the risk of failure.

Wherever you are, at home or in nursing care, make your bedroom attractive, interesting, and filled with the treasures of a lifetime.

The Crowning Days

God is sovereign over life and death. He decides the day of our death and the manner of our dying. When the times comes, it is up to Him to decide the day. How will that day come? The great majority of us will die suddenly, and for us there will be no dying process. The lesson to be learned from the sudden death of the majority is that all of us should live in readiness for death, with a last will and testament completed, with instructions to our executors, trustees, family, and friends.

Some fade away slowly. This is usually a painless gradual increase of weakness caused by the failure of one or more of our vital systems, and slipping into unconsciousness, a fading away. The age of painless dying is an age when we should not be embarrassed to seek pain relief as required.

The dying need a companion in their final hours and moments who will go all the way to the edge with them, and who will hold their hands affectionately.

There are many legitimate reasons to be afraid of dying, and these fears should not arouse guilt. These legitimate fears are: fear of pain, fear of the unknown, fear for the future of one's family, and fear of shame and embarrassment.

There is no legitimate reason to fear death itself if we understand and accept God's gift of eternal life through Jesus Christ.

The Pathway to Joy

What is the pathway to a joyful second half? Science and Christian faith both provide us with clues as we study the aging process and the life span.

We have studied the aging process in detail to understand how to extend life and how to improve it.

We have also studied the life span, especially the six segments of the second half of life.

Our purpose, in this twofold study of aging and the life span, has been to unfold the Christian pathway to joy, as defined and supported by Scripture and as confirmed by recent scientific research.

The new science of aging relates so well to Christian faith and practice. Let Christian people, workers with the elderly, and all persons in middle and older adulthood be encouraged by the joyful possibilities of the second half of life.

Bibliography

Atchley, R. C. *Social Forces in Later Life.* Belmont, California: Wadsworth Publishing Company, 1972.

Birren, J. E., ed. *Human Aging.* Vol. 1. Washington, D. C.: U. S. Government Printing Office, 1963.

Birren, J. E., and D. S. Woodruff. *Aging: Scientific Perspectives and Social Issues.* New York: Van Nostrand and Company, 1975.

Botwinick, J., and J. E. Birren. "Cognitive Processes" in Birren, *Human Aging* (above).

Campbell, A. "The American Way of Mating." *Psychology Today* 8: 37-41.

Eisdorfer, C., and C. Service. "Verbal Rote Learning and Superior Intelligence in the Aged." *Journal of Gerontology* 22: 158-161, 1967.

Erikson, E. "Growth and Crises of the Healthy Personality." *Psychological Issues,* Vol. 1, 1959.

Filer, R. N., and D. O. O'Connell. "Motivation of Aging Persons." *Journal of Gerontology* 19: 15-22, Jan. 1964.

Glen, M. "Psychological Well-Being in the Post-Parental Stage." *Journal of Marriage and the Family* 32: 105-110, 1975.

Hagestad, G. O. *Role Change and Socialization in Adulthood.* Unpublished manuscript. Pennsylvania State University, 1980.

Jung, Carl. *The Portable Jung.* New York: Viking Press, 1971.

Levinson, D. "Else Frenkel-Brunswik." *International Encyclopedia of the Social Sciences.* Vol. 5, 1968.

Levinson, D., et al. *The Seasons of a Man's Life.* New York: Alfred A. Knopf, 1978.

Neugarten, B. L. *Personality in Middle and Late Life.* New York: Atherton House, 1964.

Spieth, W. "Cardiovascular Health Status, Age, and Psychological Performance." *Journal of Gerontology* 19: 277-284, 1964.

Y Gasset, Jose Ortega, *Man and Crisis.* New York: W.W. Norton, 1958.